T0274206

Early Pregnancy Issues for the MRCOG and Beyond

Published titles in the MRCOG and Beyond series

Antenatal Disorders for the MRCOG and Beyond
by Andrew Thomson and Ian Greer

Fetal Medicine for the MRCOG and Beyond, second edition
by Alan Cameron, Janet Brennand, Lena Crichton and Janice Gibson

Gynaecological and Obstetric Pathology for the MRCOG and Beyond,
second edition *edited by Michael Wells, C Hilary Buckley and Harold Fox,
with a chapter on cervical cytology by John Smith*

Gynaecological Oncology for the MRCOG and Beyond,
second edition *edited by Nigel Acheson and David Luesley*

Gynaecological Urology for the MRCOG and Beyond
by Simon Jackson, Meghana Pandit and Alexandra Blackwell

Haemorrhage and Thrombosis for the MRCOG and Beyond *edited by
Anne Harper*

Intrapartum Care for the MRCOG and Beyond, second edition *by
Thomas F Baskett and Sabaratnam Arulkumaran, with a chapter on neonatal resuscitation by Gareth J Richards and a chapter on perinatal loss
by Austin Ugwumadu and Melanie O'Byrne*

Management of Infertility for the MRCOG and Beyond, second
edition *edited by Siladitya Bhattacharya and Mark Hamilton*

Medical Genetics for the MRCOG and Beyond *by Michael Connor*

Menopause for the MRCOG and Beyond, second edition
by Margaret Rees

Menstrual Problems for the MRCOG *by Mary Ann Lumsden,
Jane Norman and Hilary Critchley*

Neonatology for the MRCOG *by Peter Dear and Simon Newell*

Paediatric and Adolescent Gynaecology for the MRCOG
and Beyond, second edition *by Anne Garden, Mary Hernan
and Joanne Topping*

Psychological Disorders in Obstetrics and Gynaecology
for the MRCOG and Beyond *by Khaled MK Ismail, Ilana Crome
and PM Shaughn O'Brien*

Reproductive Endocrinology for the MRCOG and Beyond, second
edition *edited by Adam Balen*

The MRCOG: A Guide to the Examination *edited by William Ledger*

Early Pregnancy Issues for the MRCOG and Beyond

Geeta Kumar and Bidyut Kumar

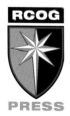

A machine-readable catalogue record for this publication is available from the British Library [www.bl.uk/catalogue/listings.html]

ISBN 978-1-906985-45-5

Published by the **RCOG Press** at the
Royal College of Obstetricians and Gynaecologists
27 Sussex Place, Regent's Park
London NW1 4RG

Registered Charity No. 213280

Cover image: Magnified view of the haemorrhagic corpus luteum demonstrating typical ultrasound scan features

RCOG Press Editor: Claire Dunn
Index: Cath Topliff
Design and typesetting: FiSH Books, London
Printed by Latimer Trend and Co. Ltd, Estover Road, Plymouth PL6 7PL

Contents

Dedication and acknowledgement

Dedicated to our parents, whose love and inspiration always guides us in the right direction and to Dona, our daughter, who continues to be a constant source of delight and joy in our lives.

We express our sincere thanks to the staff at John Spalding library, Wrexham Medical Institute for their untiring help and support in preparing this manuscript.

Geeta Kumar and Bidyut Kumar
July 2011

About the authors

Geeta Kumar FRCOG
Consultant Obstetrician and Gynaecologist
Betsi Cadwaladr University Health Board
Wrexham Maelor Hospital
Wrexham
UK

Bidyut Kumar FRCOG
Consultant Obstetrician and Gynaecologist
Betsi Cadwaladr University Health Board
Wrexham Maelor Hospital
Wrexham
UK

With contributions to the chapters on miscarriage, recurrent miscarriage and abdominal and pelvic pain in early pregnancy from:

Julia Alcide MRCOG
Consultant Obstetrician and Gynaecologist
Furness General Hospital
Barrow-in-Furness
Cumbria
UK

Abbreviations

βhCG	beta human chorionic gonadotrophin
CHM	complete hydatidiform mole
CI	confidence interval
CRL	crown–rump length
DCDA	dichorionic–diamniotic
DHEAS	dehydroepiandrosterone sulphate
DHT	dihydrotestosterone
EDD	estimated delivery date
EPAU	early pregnancy assessment unit
ERPC	evacuation of retained products of conception
ESHRE	European Society for Human Reproduction and Embryology
FVL	factor V Leiden
GFR	glomerular filtration rate
GTD	gestational trophoblastic disease
GYN	gestational trophoblastic neoplasia
hCG	human chorionic gonadotrophin
HLA	human leucocyte antigen
hPL	human placental lactogen
iu	international units
IVF	in vitro fertilisation
LH	luteinising hormone
LMP	last menstrual period
MIS	müllerian inhibiting substance
NK	natural killer
NICE	National Institute for Health and Clinical Excellence

NT	nuchal translucency
OHSS	ovarian hyperstimulation syndrome
PHM	partial hydatidiform mole
PSTT	placental site trophoblastic tumour
RhD	rhesus D antigen
SRY	sex-determining region of the Y chromosome
TORCH	toxoplasmosis, other (congenital syphilis and viruses), rubella, cytomegalovirus and herpes simplex virus
TRH	thyrotrophin-releasing hormone
TSH	thyroid-stimulating hormone
TVS	transvaginal ultrasound scan
UTI	urinary tract infection
WHO	World Health Organization

Preface

The emergence of early pregnancy units into clinical practice demands educational support and the development of clear guidelines. For the inquisitive trainee, the array of information portals, both paper and electronic, can be bewildering leading to initial confusion about where to start.

This book provides a useful vade mecum that allows a ready and accurate reference source as well as encouraging more complex reading and critical analysis for those that aspire to improved practice. This compendium represents an excellent primer while providing a solid foundation from where to start.

It makes another useful addition to a burgeoning series.

Roy G Farquharson MD FRCOG
Liverpool
November 2011

1 Embryogenesis and physiology

The average duration of pregnancy is 266 days (38 weeks) after ovulation or 280 days (40 weeks) after the first day of the last menstrual period (LMP). This equates to a period of just over 9 calendar months. Traditionally, the age of a pregnancy has been calculated from the first day of the LMP but it is easy to appreciate that this cannot be the same as the age of the embryo or the fetus, as conception does not occur until after ovulation has taken place: about 14 days after the LMP. Those involved with in vitro fertilisation usually refer to the age of embryo as being equivalent to the number of days elapsed since fertilisation and this is commonly referred to as 'gestational days'. Thus, a traditionally defined 10-week pregnancy is equivalent to 56 gestational days. This concept is important to the understanding of timing of development of the embryo which, in turn, can explain the effects of certain teratogens on different embryonic or fetal structures. The embryo changes to a fetus 10 weeks after the LMP: at 56 gestational days (8 weeks) (Table 1.1). This is an important transition because the vast majority of the adult bodily structures are recognisable by the end of the embryonic stage.

Part of the urogenital tract develops from the primitive gut tube, which also gives rise to many other organs, the most important of which are:

- the thyroid and pituitary glands
- the lungs
- the pancreas
- the bile ducts and gall bladder
- the urogenital system.

During the third week, the three primary germ layers form: the ectoderm, mesoderm and endoderm. These germ layers eventually give rise to the formation of different body organs. The intraembryonic mesoderm has four subdivisions: cardiogenic mesoderm, paraxial

Table 1.1 Chronology of development of the important embryonic structures (adapted from *Larsen's Human Embryology*, 4th ed., Schoenwolf GC, Bleyl SB, Brauer PR, Francis-West PH. Copyright Churchill Livingstone 2009)

Gestational days	Salient developmental features
1	Fertilisation
2–6	Embryo transported along the fallopian tube and becomes attached to endometrium around day 6
7–12	Blastocyst fully implanted; cells of the trophoblast produce human chorionic gonadotrophin, which supports the corpus luteum and thus maintains the supply of progesterone
16	Notochordal process forms; notochord forms the nucleus pulposus at the centre of the vertebral disc
18	Neural plate and neural groove form; the broad cranial end of neural plate gives rise to the brain and the narrower caudal portion forms the spinal cord; the neural plate folds during the 4th week to form the neural tube, the precursor of the central nervous system
End of 3rd week	The embryo is a flat, ovoid, trilaminar disc; during the 4th week it grows rapidly in length and undergoes a process of folding that generates the recognisable vertebrate body form. The outer layer is the ectoderm (future skin) which covers the entire outer surface of the embryo, except in the umbilical region where the yolk sac and connecting stalk emerge. The innermost layer is the endodermal primary gut tube. Separating the ectoderm and endoderm is a layer of mesoderm that contains the coelom. Failure of the ventral body wall to form properly during body folding results in anterior abdominal wall defects, the most common of which are omphalocele and gastroschisis
20	Vasculature begins to develop in embryonic disc; primitive heart tube forming; condensation of mesoderm, called somites, form between day 20 and day 30. Somites give rise to most of the axial skeleton including the vertebral column and part of the occipital bone of the skull
22	Neural folds begin to fuse; myocardium forms and heart begins to pump. The five pairs of pharyngeal arches start forming in a craniocaudal succession
24	Cranial neuropore closes. Failure of closure leads to anencephaly
26	Caudal neuropore closes. Failure of closure can cause neural tube defects of varying degree. Upper limb buds form
28	Septum primum begins to form in heart; ureteric buds form; lower limb buds form
29	Last of the pharyngeal arches formed
32	Cerebral hemispheres become visible
37	Muscular ventricular septum begins to form
44	Skeletal ossification begins
52	Pericardioperitoneal canals close; hands and feet rotate toward midline
77–84	Corpus luteum involutes and placenta begins to secrete large amounts of progesterone; corpus luteum becomes corpus albicans

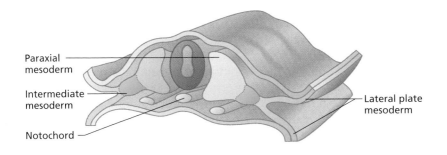

Paraxial mesoderm

Intermediate mesoderm

Notochord

Lateral plate mesoderm

Figure 1.1 Components of the intraembryonic mesoderm (reproduced with permission from *Larsen's Human Embryology*, 4th ed., Schoenwolf GC, Bleyl SB, Brauer PR, Francis-West PH. Copyright Churchill Livingstone 2009)

mesoderm, intermediate mesoderm and lateral plate mesoderm (Figure 1.1). Of these mesodermal subdivisions, the intermediate mesoderm gives rise to nephric structures of the embryo, parts of suprarenal glands, the gonads and the genital duct system.

During embryonic development, three sets of nephric systems develop in craniocaudal succession from the intermediate mesoderm. These are called pronephros, mesonephros and metanephros. The paired primitive kidney (mesonephros) develops from the intermediate mesoderm on either side of the gut tube. The intermediate mesoderm also gives rise to a pair of small ducts called mesonephric ducts (wolffian ducts). These ducts connect the mesonephros to the ventrolateral wall of the cloaca on day 26. This region of fusion will become part of the posterior wall of the future bladder. Ureteric buds grow from the distal portion of the mesonephric ducts on about day 28. The definitive kidneys develop from the metanephros and are composed of the excretory portion and the collecting portion. The ureters and the collecting duct system of the kidneys differentiate from the ureteric bud and the excretory portion (nephrons) develop from the metanephric mesenchyme.

The primitive gonad develops from the genital ridges which develop medial to each mesonephros in the intermediate mesoderm at the level of the tenth thoracic vertebra during the 5th week. At about the 46th gestational day a second paired duct system called the paramesonephric (müllerian) duct develops parallel to the mesonephric duct. These paramesonephric ducts give rise to fallopian tubes from their cranial end and uterus and upper vagina from their fused caudal portion. The lower portion of the vagina is formed from the sinovaginal bulbs which develop from the endodermal tissue surrounding posterior urethra.

In the male embryo, the secretion of a peptide called müllerian inhibiting substance (MIS) by precursors of Sertoli cells in the testis occurs under the direction of sex-determining region of the Y chromosome (SRY). MIS causes regression of the müllerian duct. The precursors of Leydig cells produce testosterone, which stimulates development of the wolffian duct system to form the epididymis, vas deferens and seminal vesicles. Testosterone production by the embryonic testis is controlled by human chorionic gonadotrophin (hCG) produced by the placenta.

The absence of MIS in the female embryo permits the müllerian system to persist. Upon reaching the urogenital sinus, the müllerian ducts induce the formation of a vaginal plate and start fusing with each other to form the body of the uterus and upper one-third of the vagina. In the absence of testosterone, the wolffian system regresses, leaving behind a vestigial tube called Gartner's duct, which extends from the ovary to the hymen. Most of the prostate gland develops from the same primordial area of the urogenital sinus that forms the vaginal plate in the female, making the prostate a homologue of the upper vagina.

Differentiation of the primordial external genital structures into recognisably male phenotype require the presence of dihydrotestosterone (DHT). The source of DHT is testicular testosterone converted locally to DHT. In the presence of DHT, the genital folds fuse to form the penis around the elongating urethra. The labioscrotal swellings enlarge and fuse to form the scrotum. In the female the folds of the urogenital slit remain open. The posterior aspect of the urogenital sinus forms the lower two-thirds of the vagina and the anterior aspect forms the urethra. The lateral genital folds form the labia minora and the labioscrotal swellings form the labia majora. Figure 1.2 shows the embryonic differentiation of the internal genital tract into male and female gender.

The expanded caudal part of the primitive hindgut is called a cloaca, which is closed at its bottom end by the cloacal membrane. Between the 22nd and 42nd day, the cloaca is partitioned into a dorsal anorectal canal and a ventral urogenital sinus by formation of the urorectal septum (Figure 1.3). The urogenital sinus gives rise to the urinary bladder, membranous urethra and the vestibule of the vagina.

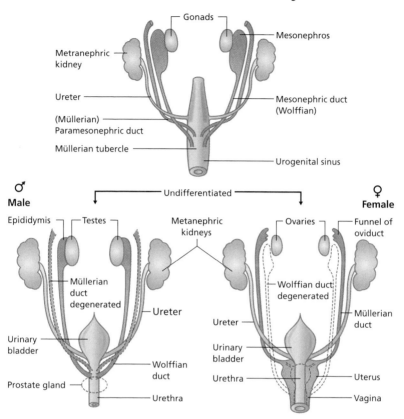

Differentiation of the male and female internal genitalia

Gonads

Mesonephros

Metranephric kidney

Ureter

Mesonephric duct (Wolffian)

(Müllerian) Paramesonephric duct

Müllerian tubercle

Urogenital sinus

♂ Male

Undifferentiated

♀ Female

Epididymis — Testes

Metanephric kidneys

Ovaries — Funnel of oviduct

Müllerian duct degenerated

Wolffian duct degenerated

Ureter

Müllerian duct

Ureter

Urinary bladder

Urinary bladder

Prostate gland

Wolffian duct

Urethra

Uterus

Urethra

Vagina

Figure 1.2 Differentiation of the internal genital tract into male and female gender (reprinted from *The Reproductive System at a Glance*, 3rd ed., LJ Heffner and DJ Schust, p. 22 (2010) with permission from John Wiley and Sons)

DESCENT OF THE GONAD

During embryonic and fetal life, the gonads in both male and female descend from their original position at the 10th thoracic level, although the testes ultimately descend much farther. In both sexes, the descent of the gonad depends on the ligamentous gubernaculum. The gubernaculum condenses during the 7th week within the subserous fascia of a longitudinal peritoneal fold on either side of the vertebral column.

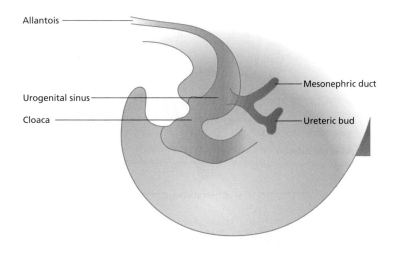

Allantois

Mesonephric duct

Urogenital sinus

Cloaca

Ureteric bud

Figure 1.3 Partitioning of the cloaca (reproduced with permission from *Larsen's Human Embryology*, 4th ed, Schoenwolf GC, Bleyl SB, Brauer PR, Francis-West PH. Copyright Churchill Livingstone 2009)

Unlike the male, the gubernaculum in the female does not swell or shorten but causes the ovaries to descend during the 3rd month and to be swept out into a peritoneal fold called the broad ligament of the uterus. This translocation occurs because, during the 7th week, the gubernaculum becomes attached to the developing müllerian ducts, where these two structures cross each other on the posterior body wall. As the müllerian ducts fuse together from the caudal ends, they sweep out the broad ligaments and simultaneously pull the ovaries into these peritoneal folds. In the absence of male hormones, the female gubernaculum remains intact and grows in step with the rest of the body. The inferior gubernaculum becomes the round ligament of the uterus connecting the fascia of the labia majora to the uterus and the superior portion becomes the ligament of the ovary, connecting the uterus to the ovary (Figure 1.4).

ASCENT OF THE KIDNEYS

The kidneys ascend to the lumbar region between the 6th and 9th weeks, following a route on either side of the dorsal aorta. The differential growth of the lumbar and sacral regions of the embryo is

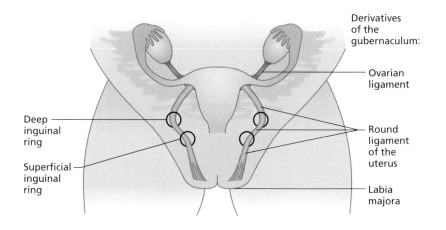

Figure 1.4 The ligament of the ovary, connecting the uterus to the ovary (reproduced with permission from *Larsen's Human Embryology*, 4th ed, Schoenwolf GC, Bleyl SB, Brauer PR, Francis-West PH. Copyright Churchill Livingstone 2009)

most likely to be responsible for such ascent. The ascending kidney is progressively vascularised by a series of arterial sprouts from the dorsal aorta and the original renal artery in the sacral region disappears. Variation in this process can result in accessory renal arteries, pelvic kidney. The right kidney usually stays at a lower level than the left kidney because of the presence of the liver on the right side (Figure 1.5).

Physiological changes in early pregnancy

In pregnancy, the female body undergoes physiological adaptations to support the developing fetus, most of which are unrelated to the actual size of the fetus.

PHYSICAL SIGNS AND SYMPTOMS OF EARLY PREGNANCY

Around the time of implantation, slight vaginal bleeding may occur and this usually takes place around 7–12 days after ovulation. Breast tenderness and tingling, especially around the nipple often occurs beginning at 4–6 weeks after the LMP. Increased breast size and vascularity are usually evident by the end of the 2nd month after LMP, caused by growth of the secretory duct system. Expression of colostrum

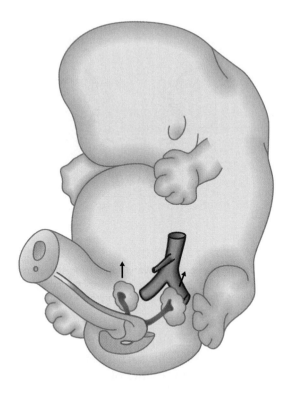

Figure 1.5 Ascent of the metanephric kidney from the sacral region to their definitive lumbar position (reproduced with permission from *Larsen's Human Embryology*, 4th ed, Schoenwolf GC, Bleyl SB, Brauer PR, Francis-West PH. Copyright Churchill Livingstone 2009)

may occur by 3 months and at this time enlargement of the sebaceous glands around the nipple (Montgomery's glands) may also be apparent. Usually beginning about 6 weeks after LMP, nausea or vomiting may occur any time of the day or night and commonly continues for 6–12 weeks or longer in some women. An increase in frequency of micturition and a feeling of fatigue are often experienced during the first trimester.

During pregnancy, the almost solid nonpregnant uterus with a cavity of 10 ml or less develops into a large, thin-walled organ, the total volume of the contents at term being 500–1000 times the original capacity. Physical signs associated with pregnancy include softening of the cervix and vagina with increased discharge of leucorrhoea (Goodell's sign), softening and increased compressibility of the lower uterine segment (Hegar's sign) and bluish purple discoloration of the vaginal mucosa, cervix and vulva (Chadwick's sign) by about 8 weeks from the LMP. Although a presumptive sign of pregnancy, Chadwick's sign is only useful in primiparous women. By 8–10 weeks, fetal heart tones can be auscultated by Doppler ultrasonography. Real-time ultrasound can detect fetal heart between 5 and 6 weeks from the LMP.

In the early second trimester, the uterus changes from a pear-shaped organ to an ovoid shape as length increases more than width. As a result, the uterine fundus may be palpable abdominally at 12 weeks after the LMP. As a result of this growth, the broad ligament and round ligament undergo tension and stretching which can give rise to sharp, painful sensations in the lower abdomen. Leucorrhoea often occurs with a thick white acidotic (pH 3.5–6.0) discharge which may contribute to inhibition of pathogenic colonisation of the vagina. The breasts become more nodular with larger, more deeply pigmented nipples and broader areola.

Increased estrogen levels may result in hyperaemic, soft, swollen gums which bleed easily. Thus, good dental care is important to avoid growth of pathogenic organisms and infection. Elevated progesterone levels decrease motility of the gastrointestinal tract, which can lead to constipation.

CARDIOVASCULAR AND HAEMODYNAMIC CHANGES

By 8 weeks, gestation systemic vasodilatation takes place and this results in a fall in systemic vascular resistance. To compensate for this, the cardiac output increases by 20%. This increase is achieved mainly by an increase in stroke volume and to a smaller extent by an increase in heart rate. The stroke volume eventually increases to about 30% above nonpregnant levels and the heart rate by about 15 beats/minute. By 28 weeks of gestation cardiac output increases by 40% from 3.5 litres/minute to about 6 litres/minute and then plateaus. This increase in cardiac output is not sufficient to counteract the fall in vascular resistance and the net effect is a slight fall in systolic blood pressure and a greater fall in diastolic blood pressure in the second trimester.

Blood volume starts rising in early pregnancy because of an increase in plasma volume and red cell volume. In pregnancy, the increase in total red cell mass is about 25%, from around 1300 ml to 1700 ml and the increase in plasma volume is about 40% from about 2600 ml to 3700 ml. Plasma volume starts rising within a few weeks after conception. This disproportionate rise in plasma volume means that there is haemodilution resulting in a physiological anaemia.

URINARY TRACT

Dilatation of the pelvicalyceal system of maternal kidney and ureters can be seen as early as the first trimester. In most cases, these changes are more pronounced on the right side, probably owing to the fact that the right ovarian vein crosses in front of the ureter on the right side but runs parallel to the ureter on the left side. In addition, the left ureter may be protected by the descending colon. Soon after conception, the glomerular filtration rate (GFR) and effective renal plasma flow increases and eventually rises by about 50% in pregnancy. The increased GFR leads to increased renal clearance of urinary constituents, in particular urea and uric acid, both of which decrease considerably during the first trimester of pregnancy. The increased filtered load as a result of increase in GFR exceeds the absorptive capacity of the renal tubules such that glucose excretion in urine increases soon after conception and many healthy pregnant women develop glycosuria detectable on urinalysis. Thus, glycosuria does not provide reliable information regarding glucose metabolism during pregnancy.

ENDOCRINE SYSTEM

Thyroid

In the late first trimester there is an increase in plasma thyroid-binding globulin. The proportion of protein-bound thyroxine increases and free thyroxine (both free T4 and free T3) falls. The feedback mechanism ensures an increase in thyrotrophin-releasing hormone (TRH) activity and thyroid-stimulating hormone (TSH) production by the anterior pituitary. This in turn leads to thyroid hyperplasia and a consequent return of free T4 and free T3 level to normal. In some cases, free T3 and T4 might show a slight fall. These changes in pregnancy make interpretation of laboratory tests difficult.

Thyroid disease during pregnancy may be associated with an increased risk of miscarriage, fetal death, preterm delivery and pre-eclampsia. There is also some evidence that subclinical hypothyroidism, defined by an increased serum level of TSH in the presence of normal levels of T4 and T3, is associated with an increased risk for some of these pregnancy complications and adverse neuropsychological development of the offspring.

Human chorionic gonadotrophin

hCG is a double-chain glycoprotein consisting of an alpha subunit chain of 147 amino acids and closely resembles luteinising hormone

(LH) secreted by the anterior pituitary and only differs by 28–30 amino acids in the terminal portion of the beta subunit. This structural difference has permitted development of radioimmunoassay specific for the beta subunit, which is now used in the diagnosis of pregnancy and management of clinical conditions such as trophoblastic disease and ovarian carcinoma. hCG is detectable in the maternal plasma around the 9th day after ovulation and is initially secreted by the blastocyst during its penetration in to the endometrial stroma and later on by the syncytiotrophoblast.

hCG is detectable in the urine and becomes detectable between the 30th and 60th day with a peak of 60–70 days. The presence of hCG in the urine is the basis of pregnancy tests on urine. The main function of hCG is to prevent the involution of corpus luteum and to stimulate the production by it of estrogen and progesterone in the first few days and weeks of pregnancy until the placenta takes over. By the 7th week the placenta produces about 50% of the total estrogen and progesterone and by the 10th week almost 90%. Removal of the corpus luteum before the 8th week may result in miscarriage.

Many studies have characterised the rise of hCG levels during normal intrauterine pregnancies, leading to the development of standard clinical policies for the management of both normal and complicated pregnancies in the first trimester. Ideally, women attending an early pregnancy assessment unit should have a positive urine-based hCG test. Modern monoclonal antibody tests can detect hCG at levels of 25 iu/litre, which corresponds to day 23 of a 28-day cycle or 9 days after conception. Both the absolute and serial levels of beta hCG is useful in the management of women with early pregnancy complications. Several authors have researched the concept of a 'discriminatory zone' of hCG, above which level an intrauterine gestation should always be visualised by transvaginal ultrasound in a normal pregnancy. Cut-off levels of hCG of 1000 iu/litre, 1500 iu/litre and 2000 iu/litre have been evaluated and different levels of hCG will give different sensitivity and specificity in the detection of ectopic pregnancy.[1] The most commonly accepted value in practice seems to be 1500 iu/litre, above which value an intrauterine pregnancy should always be visualised with transvaginal scan.[2] Serum hCG levels continuously increase in early pregnancy and, typically, by the time of the first missed period maternal circulating levels are about 100 iu/litre. Levels of hCG peak around 100 000 iu/litre between the 8th and 10th week of gestation and then decrease and remain stable at about 20 000 iu/litre.[3]

The practical use of serum levels of hCG is based on the consensus that normal intrauterine pregnancies are associated with a predictable rise in serial serum hCG values that is different from the slow rise or plateau seen with nonviable intrauterine or ectopic pregnancies. Various studies have described the rise of hCG values and the rate of increase but the suggested values have varied. One author (Kadar) established the often quoted concept of a 'doubling time' of serum hCG levels in early gestation, namely a minimum of a 66% rise in 48 hours.[4] A further study on a much larger group of women with viable pregnancies reported that rate of rise of serum hCG was different from the initial study. Defined by a 99% confidence interval (CI), the minimal rise of hCG was estimated to be 53% in 2 days. That is 99% of viable intrauterine pregnancies should have at least a 53% rise of serum hCG in 2 days.[5] It is important to note that observation of a 'normal' rise of hCG does not eliminate the possibility of miscarriage or ectopic pregnancy. Such diagnoses should be established definitively via modalities such as ultrasonography, laparoscopy or uterine evacuation.

Human placental lactogen

Human placental lactogen (hPL) is detectable in the trophoblast as early as the 3rd week and in the maternal serum at the 4th week after ovulation. Its secretion rises during pregnancy and peaks near term. hPL consists of a single polypeptide chain and its structure is very similar to human growth hormone and prolactin. It is secreted by the syncytiotrophoblast into maternal blood and the plasma concentration is proportional to the functioning placental mass that hPL promotes. The main role of hPL is regulating glucose availability for the fetus. It antagonises the action of insulin, increases maternal metabolism and use of fat as an energy substrate and reduces glucose uptake and use by maternal cells. This increases availability of glucose for transport to the fetus. Thus, hPL acts as a growth-promoting hormone, promoting fetal growth by altering maternal metabolism. Secretion of hPL is regulated by glucose; decreased serum glucose leads to increased hPL secretion and increased maternal lipolysis.

Steroidogenesis

Synthesis of steroid hormones, progesterone and the estrogens increases during pregnancy. A complex set of cooperative interactions is necessary among the mother, placenta and fetus for placental production of progesterone and estrogen. The main source of cholesterol for steroidogenesis is maternal low-density lipoproteins. The placenta lacks certain enzymes needed for production of estriol; these enzymes are present in the fetal adrenal. The fetus is the major source of specific precursors for estrogens and the mother is the major source of precursors for progesterone. Placental progesterone also serves as a precursor for fetal synthesis of corticosteroids, testosterone and androgens.

Progesterone

About 8 weeks after fertilisation, progesterone is synthesised primarily by the placenta, using maternal cholesterol and low-density lipoproteins. A fetus is not essential for placental progesterone production. In pregnancy, progesterone:

- decreases myometrial activity and irritability and constricts myometrial vessels
- decreases sensitivity of the maternal respiratory centre to carbon dioxide
- inhibits prolactin secretion
- helps to suppress maternal immunological responses to fetal antigens, thereby preventing rejection of the fetus
- relaxes smooth muscle in the gastrointestinal and urinary systems
- increases basal body temperature
- increases sodium and chloride excretion.

The most important role of progesterone in the fetus is to serve as the substrate pool for fetal adrenal gland production of glucocorticoids and mineralocorticoids. The fetal adrenal gland lacks the 3-beta hydroxylase dehydrogenase, 4-5 isomerase system necessary for the synthesis of some important corticosteroids. Thus, the fetus uses progesterone substrate from the placenta to accomplish this.

Estrogens

Estrone, estradiol and estriol are the three main estrogens. In the nonpregnant woman, estriol is derived from estradiol and estrone, whereas in pregnancy it is synthesised by the fetoplacental unit. The fetal liver and suprarenal glands are important in estriol production and estriol is a direct measure of fetal wellbeing. Approximately 90% of the precursors for estriol are derived from the fetus. The primary source of estriol precursors is dehydroepiandrosterone sulphate (DHEAS) which originates in the fetal adrenal gland under stimulation by fetal adrenocorticotropic hormone. DHEAS is hydroxylated in the fetal liver and further metabolised by the placenta to form estriol. Estriol is secreted by the placenta into maternal circulation and eventually excreted in maternal urine. Maternal serum and urinary estriol levels rise rapidly during early pregnancy, more slowly between 24 and 32 weeks and then increase rapidly again in the last 6 weeks.

Key points

- The actual age of the embryo is equal to the number of days elapsed since fertilisation, which is about 14 days less than the gestational age calculated from the date of the last menstrual period.
- Knowledge of early embryogenesis is important in understanding the origin of congenital anomalies of the fetus.
- Physiological changes in early pregnancy can cause difficulty in identifying certain pathological conditions in pregnancy.

References

1. Condous G, Kirk E, Lu C, Van Huffel S, Gevaert O, De Moor B, et al. Diagnostic accuracy of varying discriminatory zones for the prediction of ectopic pregnancy in women with a pregnancy of unknown location. *Ultrasound Obstet Gynecol* 2005;26:770–5.
2. Jones K, Pearce C. Organizing an acute gynaecology service; equipment, setup and a brief review of the likely conditions that are managed in the unit. *Best Pract Res Clin Obstet Gynaecol* 2009;23(4):427–38.
3. Chung K, Allen R. The use of serial human chorionic gonadotropin levels to establish a viable or a nonviable pregnancy. *Semin Reprod Med* 2008;26:383–90.
4. Kadar N, Caldwell BV, Romero RA. A method of screening for ectopic pregnancy and its indications. *Obstet Gynecol* 1981;58:162–6.
5. Barnhart KT, Sammel MD, Rinaudo PF, Zhou L, Hummel AC, Guo W. Symptomatic patients with an early viable intrauterine pregnancy; HCG curves redefined. *Obstet Gynecol* 2004;104:50–5.

2   Miscarriage

Miscarriage is the most common early pregnancy complication, with an incidence of approximately 15–20% of all clinically recognised pregnancies. The vast majority of miscarriages occur before 12 weeks of gestation and less than 5% occur after detection of fetal heart activity.[1] Miscarriage is not only associated with significant psychological distress for the woman and her partner but also contributes towards a serious burden for healthcare providers. There is good evidence to suggest that appropriate counselling and support to women after miscarriage offers significant beneficial effects.

Definition of miscarriage

Miscarriage is generally defined in the UK as the loss of an intrauterine pregnancy before 24 completed weeks of gestation.[2] The World Health Organization (WHO) defines miscarriage as 'the expulsion from its mother of an embryo or fetus weighing 500 g or less, corresponding to a gestational age of up to 20 completed weeks of gestation with no signs of life'.[3]

With advances in neonatal intensive care and the survival of some babies born before 24 weeks, the WHO definition seems to be the preferred one for most international epidemiological studies.

Miscarriage is traditionally classed as first-trimester or early miscarriage when it occurs before 12 weeks of gestation and as second- or mid-trimester or late miscarriage between 12 and 24 weeks of gestation.

Terminology

Medical terminology for miscarriage has changed over time and it is now widely accepted that the term 'abortion' should be avoided when describing spontaneous miscarriage. The European Society for Human Reproduction and Embryology (ESHRE) special interest group for early pregnancy has published recommendations for appropriate terminology to be used in relation to miscarriage to ensure clarity and consistency (Table 2.1).[2]

Table 2.1. Revised nomenclature (ESHRE): RCOG Green-top Guideline No 25, 2006[2]

Term	Definition
Biochemical pregnancy loss	Pregnancy not located on scan
Empty sac	Gestation sac with absent or minimal structures
Fetal loss	Previously seen intrauterine pregnancy with subsequent loss of fetal heart activity
Early pregnancy loss or delayed miscarriage	Confirmed empty sac or sac with fetus but no fetal heart activity less than 12 weeks
Late pregnancy loss	Loss of fetal heart activity after 12 weeks
Pregnancy of unknown location	Positive pregnancy test with no identifiable pregnancy on scan

Aetiology

The exact aetiology of miscarriage remains poorly understood but various pathogenic factors and risk factors have been identified by researchers. Box 2.1 summarises the possible causes of spontaneous miscarriage in the first and second trimesters.

FETAL CHROMOSOMAL DISORDERS

Almost 50% of clinically recognised first-trimester pregnancy losses can be apportioned to fetal chromosomal disorders, with 50% of these being autosomal trisomies, 20% 45XO monosomy, 20% polyploidy and 10% being other chromosomal abnormalities.[4] The incidence of chromosomal disorder as an identifiable cause of miscarriage decreases as pregnancy advances to about 15–20% in the second trimester.

IMMUNOLOGICAL FACTORS

Autoimmune disorders

Nearly 15% of women undergoing investigations for recurrent miscarriage are found to be positive for lupus anticoagulant or antiphospholipid antibodies.[5] In this group of women, treatment with low-dose aspirin and/or low-molecular-weight heparin has been found to be effective.

Alloimmune disorders

It has been postulated that miscarriage might occur as a result of maternal immunological rejection of fetal trophoblastic cells. However, immunisation of women against paternally derived antigens to help prevent fetal rejection and miscarriage has not met with any success.[5]

BOX 2.1 POSSIBLE CAUSES OF SPONTANEOUS MISCARRIAGE

FIRST TRIMESTER

- Chromosomal disorders (50% of miscarriages):
  - trisomies (50%)
  - triploidies (20%)
  - monosomy X (20%)
  - others (10%)
- Other factors:
  - previous history of miscarriages
  - antiphospholipid syndrome
  - uncontrolled maternal medical conditions
  - maternal infections
  - listeria
  - toxoplasmosis
  - malaria
  - herpes zoster
  - rubella
- Increasing maternal age: women over 40 years of age have a five-fold increase in miscarriage rates compared with women aged 25–29 years
- Multiple pregnancy
- High levels of maternal alcohol and caffeine consumption

MID-TRIMESTER

- Infection:
  - chorioamnionitis
  - maternal systemic infections
- Cervical weakness
- Stuctural uterine abnormality
- Thrombophilia
- Genetic causes such as trisomies 13, 18, 21, monosomy X and sex chromosomal abnormalities

ENDOCRINE CAUSES

Luteal-phase dysfunction resulting in inadequate progesterone levels has long been postulated as a possible cause for miscarriage. However, the role of progesterone in the prevention of miscarriage, especially sporadic miscarriage, remains unproven.

The incidence of miscarriage is found to be higher in women with polycystic ovary disease. This is possibly explained by high levels of luteinising hormone in the follicular phase of the menstrual cycle.[5]

There is some evidence to indicate that women with poorly controlled diabetes mellitus are more likely to suffer miscarriage when compared with those with good glycaemic control. There is, however, no definite link between thyroid dysfunction and miscarriage.[5]

INFECTION

High pyrexia from any cause may be associated with spontaneous fetal loss. Viral infections such as rubella and cytomegalovirus or bacterial infections such as malaria have all been linked with miscarriage.

UTERINE STRUCTURAL ABNORMALITIES

Bicornuate uterus, septate uterus or uterine fibroids may be occasionally associated with miscarriage.

EPIDEMIOLOGICAL FACTORS

While maternal heavy alcohol consumption, cigarette smoking and caffeine consumption have been associated with increased risk of spontaneous miscarriage, the association of miscarriage with employment involving the use of video display terminals and anaesthetic gases remains unproven. High body mass index remains an independent risk factor for both spontaneous and recurrent miscarriage.

IDIOPATHIC FACTORS

Fifty percent of miscarriages are sporadic with no recurrent identifiable cause.

Clinical diagnosis of miscarriage (Figure 2.1)

Miscarriage usually presents with vaginal bleeding and lower abdominal pain. Based on these symptoms and clinical examination findings, miscarriage can be classed as:

- **threatened** – characterised by vaginal bleeding with a closed internal os and presumed continuing pregnancy. Diagnosis is confirmed by ultrasound scan detection of a viable pregnancy. Over 90% of women in whom fetal heart activity is detected at 8 weeks will continue the pregnancy and can be reassured.[1]
- **inevitable** – presenting with vaginal bleeding and open cervical os with the pregnancy still retained within the uterine cavity.
- **incomplete** – typically presenting with bleeding and pain and open cervical os. Some products of conception remain inside the uterus or may even lie within the cervix producing a profound vagal response.
- **missed miscarriage** – associated with no symptoms or minimal vaginal bleed or brownish loss. There may be loss of pregnancy symptoms and failure of the uterus to grow. Cervical os remains closed.
- **complete miscarriage** – there is initially bleeding with pain followed by spontaneous resolution of symptoms after expulsion of products of conception. Cervical os is usually closed on examination.
- **septic miscarriage** –miscarriage complicated by genital tract infection. Common causative organisms are *Escherischia coli*, bacteroides, Streptococcus and *Clostridium welchi*. Septic miscarriage is often associated with pain, vaginal bleeding, fever and malaise.

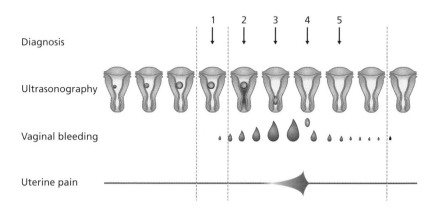

Figure 2.1 Clinical and ultrasound features of a miscarriage (published in *Clinical Obstetrics and Gynaecology*, 2nd ed., Magowan BA, Owen P, Drife J, 'Miscarriage' p. 97–102. Copyright Elsevier 2009.)[5]

Diagnosis

Establishing a correct diagnosis is vital in the management of women with spontaneous miscarriage. In this regard, history and clinical examination alone do not always suffice and ultrasound scanning remains the most reliable tool for establishing a diagnosis. Ultrasound helps to provide maternal reassurance, where fetal cardiac activity is seen and is pivotal in the assessment of early pregnancy complications.[6] A transvaginal scan (TVS) can confirm intrauterine pregnancy at an earlier gestational age compared with transabdominal ultrasound and is well accepted by the majority of women.

Various ultrasound criteria have been described for establishing a correct diagnosis and these have been summarised in Table 2.2. Ultrasound scanning should always be undertaken by appropriately qualified individuals and the reporting should be done in a standardised format to include the following:

- number of sacs and mean gestation sac diameter
- regularity of the outline of sac and its location
- presence of haematoma
- presence of a yolk sac
- presence of a fetal pole
- crown–rump length measurement (mm)
- presence of fetal heart pulsation
- extrauterine observations – ovaries, adnexal mass, fluid in the pouch of Douglas.

If there is any doubt about fetal viability, a repeat scan is strongly recommended and this is best performed after an interval of at least 7 days.

Diagnosis of complete miscarriage based on ultrasound scan is made on visualisation of an empty uterus or endometrial thickness less than 15 mm. It is important, however, that the diagnosis of complete miscarriage is only made when a prior intrauterine pregnancy has been confirmed by ultrasound, otherwise one should use the term 'pregnancy of unknown location' and management should be with serum human chorionic gonadotrophin (hCG) follow-up. In one study in women in whom TVS was suggestive of complete miscarriage, follow-up with serial hCG detected an underlying ectopic pregnancy in 5.9% of cases.[8]

Table 2.2 Transvaginal scan criteria for diagnosis of miscarriage[2,4,7*]

Diagnostic term	Ultrasound criteria
Empty sac (Figure 2.2)	Gestation sac with a mean sac diameter greater than or equal to 25 mm with no visible embryo or yolk sac
Embryonic or fetal loss	Embryo with crown rump length of more than or equal to 7 mm with no visible cardiac activity
	Or
	Initial visualisation of an embryo or fetus with visible cardiac activity, followed by repeat transvaginal ultrasound scan (TVS) showing an absence of cardiac activity
Early pregnancy loss or delayed miscarriage (Figure 2.3)	Initial visualisation of an embryo or fetus with visible cardiac activity, followed by repeat TVS showing an absence of cardiac activity
	Or
	The presence of an embryo of less than 7 mm in which cardiac activity is not visible when repeat scan is performed after at least 7 days (may also be referred to as an embryonic loss)
	Or
	The presence of an intrauterine gestation sac of less than 25 mm in which an embryo does not become visible when repeat scan is performed after at least 7 days (may also be referred to as an empty sac)
Incomplete miscarriage (Figure 2.4)	Irregular heterogeneous echoes within the endometrial cavity
Complete miscarriage	The ultrasound finding of an empty uterus after initial visualisation of an intrauterine gestation sac (with or without an embryo)
	Or
	The ultrasound finding of an empty uterus in association with a positive pregnancy test, followed by rapid decrease in serum hCG levels (more appropriately termed failed pregnancy of unknown location as a failed ectopic pregnancy cannot be ruled out)

* Revised definition of miscarriage based on addendum to RCOG Green-top Guideline No. 25, *The Management of Early Pregnancy Loss*. RCOG e-notice sent 20 October 2011.

Management

The majority of women who miscarry are referred to hospital. Dedicated early pregnancy assessment units are best placed for optimal

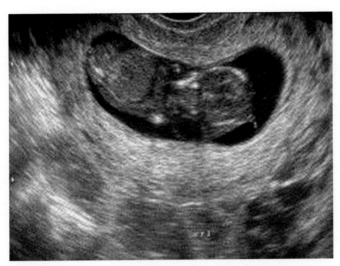

Figure 2.2 Transvaginal ultrasound scan of an intrauterine gestation sac with a mean sac diameter of greater than 20 mm (empty sac or delayed miscarriage) (reprinted from *Best Practice and Research: Clinical Obstetrics and Gynaecology* 23 (4), Bottomley C and Bourne T, Diagnosing miscarriage, 463–77, 2009, with permission from Elsevier)[4]

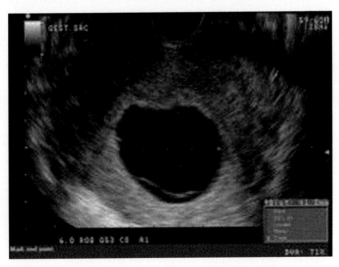

Figure 2.3 Transvaginal ultrasound scan of an intrauterine gestation sac containing an embryo of greater than 6 mm with no visible cardiac activity (delayed miscarriage or early pregnancy loss); this image also shows that the fetus has a cystic hygroma (reprinted from *Best Practice and Research: Clinical Obstetrics and Gynaecology* 23 (4), Bottomley C and Bourne T, Diagnosing miscarriage, 463–77, 2009, with permission from Elsevier)[4]

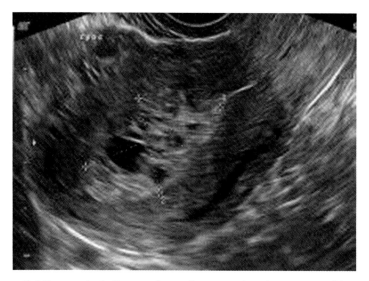

Figure 2.4 Transvaginal ultrasound scan demonstrating the presence of irregular heterogenous echoes within the endometrial cavity (incomplete miscarriage) (reprinted from *Best Practice and Research: Clinical Obstetrics and Gynaecology* 23 (4), Bottomley C and Bourne T, Diagnosing miscarriage, 463–77, 2009, with permission from Elsevier)[4]

management of miscarriage. It is recommended that women should be offered the choice of expectant, medical or surgical management of miscarriage as clinically appropriate. In one study, almost 89% of women expressed their preference for a particular method of management after being diagnosed with miscarriage.[9] Improved patient satisfaction rates are inevitable when women are allowed to make an informed choice about their miscarriage management. The risk of infection (around 2–3%) and subsequent fertility were found to be similar, with all three treatment modalities in a multicentre randomised controlled study.[10,11]

As discussed, it is agreed by a majority of clinicians that the absence of tissue in the uterine cavity or products of conception less than 15 mm in maximum anteroposterior diameter on ultrasound scan requires no intervention. With retained products measuring between 15 and 50 mm, women may be considered for medical or expectant management. Miscarriages with retained products of more than 50 mm may be better managed by surgical evacuation. Those presenting with vaginal bleeding and those who have detectable intervillous pulsatile blood flow on ultrasound scan are more likely to report successful outcome after expectant management.[12]

EXPECTANT MANAGEMENT

Expectant or conservative management involves watchful waiting for the pregnancy to miscarry and resolve spontaneously without medical or surgical intervention. Although the majority of women (70%) tend to miscarry in the first 2 weeks, this may take as long as 6–8 weeks. Factors favourable for the successful expectant treatment include a diagnosis of incomplete miscarriage (84%) compared with missed miscarriage (56%), vaginal bleeding at presentation, low serum biochemical markers (βhCG, progesterone) and pulsatile intravillous blood flow on scan.[12,13] It is important that women managed expectantly have rapid access to surgical treatment if necessary. While conservative management can be continued for those women who opt for it for as long as they are willing and there are no signs of infection or any other contraindications (see below), prolonged follow-up (sometimes 6–8 weeks) is known to yield higher success rates. Appropriate counselling and reassurance that during the course of expectant management, if they change their mind and request surgical evacuation, this could be arranged without undue delay has been found to increase the uptake of this choice of management.[14]

BENEFITS

- Avoids surgical procedure and its associated risks including risks of anaesthesia
- Allows women to continue their near-normal routine
- More acceptable to some women

RISKS

- May have more prolonged bleeding or infection
- Timescale and outcome are not always predictable
- 21–59% may need surgical evacuation

CONTRAINDICATIONS

- Heavy vaginal bleeding or haemodynamic instability
- Anaemia
- Signs of infection (pyrexia greater than 37.5°C, foul-smelling discharge, tachycardia)

MEDICAL MANAGEMENT

Medical management is successful in 70–96% of incomplete miscarriages and 52–92% of delayed miscarriages. Various agents such as hypertonic fluids, oxytocin and prostaglandins have been used for medical management of miscarriage but the prostaglandin analogue misoprostol and gemeprost are deemed to be very potent and have been used successfully in the UK for this purpose. Gemeprost (prostaglandin E_1) requires refridgeration while misoprostol remains stable at room temperature and is relatively cheaper. Several different regimens have been described in the literature with comparable success rates.

Medical management in incomplete miscarriage

Success rates varying from as low as 13% to a high of 95.3% have been reported in the literature, with the use of a single dose of 400 micrograms of oral misoprostol for management of miscarriage with retained products of conception in the first trimester of pregnancy. Others have used oral or vaginal misoprostol in divided doses of 400 micrograms every 4 hours up to 1.2 mg/day or vaginal gemeprost up to a maximum of 5 mg with similar results. Vaginal administration of prostaglandins is associated with lesser adverse effects of nausea and diarrhoea.

Medical management in missed or delayed miscarriage

With delayed miscarriage, if there is no bleeding, it is usual to give mifepristone 200 mg orally 48 hours before administering misoprostol in doses of 400 micrograms orally or vaginally initially and 400 micrograms 4 hours later orally or vaginally if the products are not expelled. In these cases, use of the anti-progestogen mifepristone helps with cervical ripening and placental separation. Fifty percent of women will start to miscarry after taking mifepristone. The morbidity among women treated medically is lower than those treated surgically (1.7% compared with 6.6%).[15] Success rates of 92–96% have been observed in pregnancies less than 10 weeks or with a mean sac diameter less than 24 mm.[16] A Cochrane review to assess the efficacy of various different treatment regimens for medical management of first-trimester miscarriage confirmed that vaginal misoprostol was more effective compared with placebo in achieving complete miscarriage within 24 hours and this therefore reduced the need for surgical intervention.[17]

BENEFITS

- Avoids the risks associated with surgery and anaesthesia
- Faster resolution compared with expectant management

RISKS

- Greater analgesic needs
- More vaginal bleeding
- Possible need for surgical evacuation in up to 30–40% of cases
- Gastrointestinal adverse effects of medications: diarrhoea, vomiting etc

CONTRAINDICATIONS (ABSOLUTE)

- Heavy vaginal bleeding and/or haemodynamic instability
- Anaemia (if in doubt, check haemoglobin and if less than 10 g/dl diagnose anaemia)
- Signs of infection (pyrexia greater than 37.5°C, tachycardia, foul-smelling vaginal discharge)
- Suspected ectopic pregnancy
- Adrenal insufficiency
- Long-term glucocorticoid therapy
- Haemoglobinopathies or anticoagulant therapy
- Known allergy to mifepristone or prostaglandin
- Porphyria
- Smokers over 35 years of age

CONTRAINDICATIONS (RELATIVE)

- Hypertension
- Severe asthma

SURGICAL MANAGEMENT

Surgical evacuation of retained products of conception (ERPC) involves dilatation of the cervix and removal of the products of conception through suction or curettage. Suction evacuation is preferable to sharp curettage as it is quicker, less painful and is associated with less blood loss and complications such as haemorrhage, sepsis, intrauterine adhesions, amenorrhoea and subfertility.[18] Preoperative priming with 400 micrograms of misoprostol administered either vaginally or orally 3 hours before ERPC is known to be associated with a reduced risk of cervical trauma, as dilatation is made easier.[19] Success rates of 95–100% are reported for surgical uterine evacuation of retained pregnancy products. The disadvantages of this method include complications of general anaesthesia and traumatic injuries such as uterine perforation and cervical trauma. Although ERPC is traditionally performed under general anaesthesia in UK, there is a growing evidence for the use of local anaesthesia in the form of a paracervical block and conscious sedation with agents such as midazolam for this procedure.[20] Up to 5/100 women may need repeat evacuation following surgical management of miscarriage and no specific risk factors for failed surgical evacuation have been documented.[21]

BENEFITS

- Planned and predictable treatment
- Less bleeding
- High success rates

RISKS

- Need for anaesthesia
- Risk of complications such as uterine perforation and cervical trauma
- Intrauterine adhesions

Histological examination

The RCOG, in its guideline, *The Management of Early Pregnancy Loss*, recommends that all tissue obtained from surgical evacuation should be sent for histological examination to help diagnose molar pregnancy and to exclude ectopic pregnancy by detection of chorionic tissue in the retained products of conception.[2] It is vital that the disposal of embryonic or fetal remains is performed in a sensitive manner, irrespective of how the loss occurred. Good practice guidance has been developed by the RCOG to help clinicians in this field.[22] All units should ensure that information regarding fetal tissue disposal is freely available and clear to all, taking into account any particular needs of the woman or couple, such as literacy skills and language. Any personal, religious or cultural needs relating to the disposal of the fetal tissue should be met wherever possible and should be documented in the woman's medical notes. Some women or couples may not wish to receive information about, or take part in, the disposal of the fetal tissues and these wishes should be respected.

Immunoprophylaxis

RCOG guidance on immunoprophylaxis recommends:

- Anti-D immunoglobulin should be given to all non-sensitised women who are RhD negative who have a spontaneous complete or incomplete miscarriage at or after 12^{+0} weeks of gestation.
- Anti-D is not required for spontaneous miscarriage before 12^{+0} weeks of gestation provided there is no uterine instrumentation.
- Anti-D should be administered to non-sensitised women who are RhD negative undergoing surgical evacuation of the uterus, regardless of gestation.
- Anti-D should be considered for non-sensitised women who are RhD negative who are undergoing medical evacuation of the uterus, regardless of gestation.
- Anti-D should be given to all non-sensitised women who are RhD negative with threatened miscarriage after 12^{+0} weeks of gestation. Women who continue to have intermittent vaginal bleeding after 12^{+0} weeks of gestation should be given anti-D at 6-weekly intervals.
- Anti-D should be considered in non-sensitised women who are RhD negative if there is heavy or repeated bleeding or associated abdominal pain as gestation approaches 12^{+0} weeks.

When indicated, anti-D immunoglobulin is administered in a dose of 250 iu up to 19^{+6} weeks of gestation and in a dose of 500 iu thereafter. The Kleihauer test to assess the size of the fetomaternal haemorrhage should be performed when anti-D immunoglobulin is given at or after 20^{+0} weeks of gestation.[23]

Psychological factors and counselling

Reactions to miscarriage tend to be variable and many women and their partners experience intense grief similar to a late pregnancy loss. Up to 50% of women suffer some form of psychological effect such as anxiety and depression. It is important to treat women and their families sensitively during this period and not to trivialise the event. Clear information and understanding can help couples adjust to the loss and restore some feeling of control. Information in verbal and written form with contact numbers for the early pregnancy unit and voluntary organisations such as the Miscarriage Association should be provided (Box 2.2). Women should be given time to help reach a decision regarding management and in such cases expectant management is suitable for the interim period.

BOX 2.2 MISCARRIAGE SUPPORT GROUP INFORMATION

Early Pregnancy Information Centre
Association of Early Pregnancy Units
Website: www.earlypregnancy.org.uk

Miscarriage Association (registered charity No: 1076829)
c/o Clayton Hospital, Northgate, Wakefield,
West Yorkshire WF1 3JS.
Tel: 01924 200799;
website: www.miscarriageassociation.org.uk

Child Bereavement Charity
The Saunderton Estate, Wycombe Road, Saunderton,
Buckinghamshire, HP14 4BF.
Tel. 01494 568900;
website: www.childbereavement.org.uk/contact_us

Royal College of Obstetricians and Gynaecologists
Website: www.rcog.org.uk

The Ectopic Pregnancy Trust
Website: www.ectopicpregnancy.org.uk

Key points

- Miscarriage is the most common early pregnancy complication and remains a significant burden for the woman, her family and health-care professionals.
- Management of miscarriage can be expectant, medical or surgical and should reflect the wishes of the woman.

- Dedicated early pregnancy assessment units are best placed to provide optimal evidence-based management of these women.
- Access to formal counselling facilities plays a vital role in the holistic management of this distressing condition.

References

1. Brigham S, Conlon C, Farquharson RG. A longitudinal study of pregnancy outcome following idiopathic recurrent miscarriage. *Hum Reprod* 1999;14:2868–71.
2. Royal College of Obstetricians and Gynaecologists. *The Management of Early Pregnancy Loss*. Green-top Guideline No. 25. London: RCOG; 2006. [www.rcog.org.uk/womens-health/clinical-guidance/management-early-pregnancy-loss-green-top-25].
3. World Health Organization. Recommended definitions, terminology and format for statistical tables related to the perinatal period. *Acta Obstet Gynecol Scand* 1977;56:247–53.
4. Bottomley C, Bourne T. Diagnosing miscarriage. *Best Pract Res Clin Obstet Gynaecol* 2009;23:463–77.
5. Owen P. Miscarriage. In: Magowan BA, Owen P, Drife J. *Clinical Obstetrics and Gynaecology*. 2nd ed. London: Saunders; 2009. p. 97–102.
6. Jauniaux E, Kaminopetros P, El-Rafaey H. Early pregnancy loss. In: Rodeck CH, Whittle MJ, editors. *Fetal Medicine*. Edinburgh: Churchill Livingstone; 2009. p. 835–84.
7. Farquharson RG, Jauniaux E, Exalto N; ESHRE Special Interest Group for Early Pregnancy. Updated and revised nomenclature for description of early pregnancy events. *Hum Reprod* 2005;20:3008–11.
8. Condous G, Okaro E, Khalid A, Bourne T. Do we need to follow up complete miscarriages with serum human chorionic gonadotrophin levels? *BJOG* 2005;112:827–9.
9. Hamilton-Fairley D, Donaghy J. Surgical versus expectant management of first trimester miscarriage: a prospective observational study. In: Grudzinskas JG, O'Brien P. *Problems in Early Pregnancy: Advances in Diagnosis and Management*. London: RCOG Press; 1997. p. 277–83.
10. Trinder J, Brocklehurst P, Porter R, Read M, Vyas S, Smith L. Management of miscarriage: expectant, medical or surgical? Results of randomised controlled trial (miscarriage treatment [MIST] trial). *BMJ* 2006;332:1235–40.
11. Smith LF, Ewings PD, Quinlan C. Incidence of pregnancy after expectant, medical, or surgical management of spontaneous first trimester miscarriage: long-term follow-up of miscarriage treatment (MIST) randomised controlled trial. *BMJ* 2009;339:b3827 [doi: 10.1136/bmj.b3827].
12. Schwärzler P, Holden D, Nielsen S, Hahlin M, Sladkevicius P, Bourne TH. The conservative management of first trimester miscarriages and the use of colour Doppler sonography for patient selection. *Hum Reprod* 1999;14:1341–5.
13. Sur SD, Raine-Fenning NJ. The management of miscarriage. *Best Pract Res Clin Obstet Gynaecol* 2009;23:479–91.
14. Luise C, Jermy K, May C, Costello G, Collins WP, Bourne TH. Outcome of expectant management of spontaneous first trimester miscarriage: observational study. *BMJ* 2002;324:873–5.
15. Hinshaw HKS. Medical management of miscarriage. In: Grudzinkas TG, O'Brien PMS, editors. *Problems in Early Pregnancy: Advances in Diagnosis and Management*. London: RCOG Press; 1997. p. 284–95.
16. de Jonge ET, Makin JD, Manefeldt E, De Wet GH, Pattinson RC. Randomised clinical trial of medical evacuation and surgical curettage for incomplete miscarriage. *BMJ* 1995;311:662.

17. Neilson JP, Hickey M, Vasquez J. Medical treatment for early fetal death (less than 24 weeks). *Cochrane Database Syst Rev* 2006;(3):CD002253.
18. Forna F, Gulmezoglu AM. Surgical procedures to evacuate incomplete abortion. Cochrane database systematic review. *Cochrane Database Syst Rev* 2001;CD001993.
19. Singh K, Fong FY. Preparation of the cervix for surgical termination of pregnancy in the first trimester. *Hum Reprod Update* 2000;6:442–8.
20. Wong CYG, Ng EHY, Ngai SW, Ho PC. A randomized double blind placebo controlled study to investigate the use of conscious sedation in conjunction with paracervical block for reducing pain in termination of first trimester pregnancy by suction evacuation. *Hum Reprod* 2002;17:1222–5.
21. Royal College of Obstetricians and Gynaecologists. *Surgical Evacuation of the Uterus for Early Pregnancy Loss*. Consent Advice No. 10. London: RCOG; 2010 [www.rcog.org.uk/surgical-evacuation-uterus-early-pregnancy-loss-consent-advice-10].
22. Royal College of Obstetricians and Gynaecologists. *Disposal Following Pregnancy Loss before 24 Weeks of Gestation*. Good Practice No. 5. London: RCOG; 2005 [www.rcog.org.uk/womens-health/clinical-guidance/disposal-following-pregnancy-loss-24-weeks-gestation].
23. Royal College of Obstetricians and Gynaecologists. *The Use of Anti-D Immunoglobulin for Rhesus D Prophylaxis*. Green-top Guideline No. 22. London: RCOG; 2011 [www.rcog.org.uk/womens-health/clinical-guidance/use-anti-d-immunoglobulin-rh-prophylaxis-green-top-22].

3   Recurrent miscarriage

Recurrent miscarriage is defined as loss of three or more consecutive pregnancies. It affects 1% of all women.[1] This incidence is greater than that expected by chance alone as, based on a 10–15% risk of spontaneous miscarriage among clinically recognised pregnancies, this would be expected to be around 0.34%. So it is understandable that only a small proportion of women will be found to have an underlying aetiology identified as the cause for recurrent miscarriage. Recurrent miscarriage could be further labelled as 'primary recurrent miscarriage', where women have had no successful pregnancies, or as secondary recurrent miscarriage, where women miscarry repetitively after a successful pregnancy or pregnancies.

Aetiology

UNKNOWN OR IDIOPATHIC

Almost 50% of all recurrent miscarriages remain unexplained despite investigations. Most women who have two or three miscarriages have nothing wrong with them and this is the justification for not undertaking tests and investigations routinely before three consecutive miscarriages. Any drug treatment in this group would be empirical and the mainstay of management of these women is based upon emotional support supplemented by ultrasound scan in early pregnancy, which gives success rates of between 70% and 80%.

GENETIC AND CHROMOSOMAL

Recurrent miscarriage may be as a result of an abnormal embryo resulting from chromosomal abnormalities or structural malformations. Genetic or chromosomal factors are responsible for recurrent miscarriage in 3–5% of couples. Either the woman or her partner may have a chromosomal abnormality which they happen to repeatedly pass on to the fetus. The most common chromosomal anomaly causing recurrent miscarriages is a parental balanced reciprocal or Robertsonian translocation.[2,3] It is recommended that cytogenetic analysis should be carried out on the products of conception of the third and subsequent consecutive miscarriages and, where this reports an unbalanced chromosomal abnormality, both partners should undergo peripheral blood karyotyping. On detection of a balanced translocation, these couples should be referred to a clinical geneticist for genetic counselling. The prevalence of chromosomal anomaly tends to decrease as the number of miscarriages increases and thus, if the karyotype of the miscarried pregnancy is found to be abnormal, the prognosis for future pregnancies is known to be better. Couples need to be informed that there is a 40–50% chance of a healthy birth in future untreated pregnancies following natural conception.[4] Couples may be offered preimplantation genetic diagnosis as a treatment option in future pregnancies.[5]

ABNORMALITIES OF THE UTERUS OR CERVIX

Studies have shown an increased prevalence of uterine anomalies in women who experience recurrent late miscarriage. The prevalence of uterine abnormalities in women who suffer recurrent miscarriage ranges widely from 1.8% to 37%, reflecting the lack of consistency in the criteria used for diagnosis of these anatomical abnormalities.[6] Uterine abnormalities such as bicornuate uterus, unicornuate uterus, septate uterus or fibroid uterus may be detected on detailed ultrasound scan or hysteroscopy. Three-dimensional ultrasound appears to be more accurate at correctly diagnosing uterine anomalies than conventional ultrasound. The use of routine hysterosalpingography for detecting uterine malformations remains questionable.[1]

It is not clear whether there is any benefit in surgical correction of these abnormalities once detected, although observational studies have shown some benefit of hysteroscopic surgical correction when compared with open uterine surgery.[1]

Cervical weakness

True cervical weakness is thought to contribute to 1% of recurrent miscarriage. Unfortunately, cervical weakness or insufficiency (formerly known as incompetence) is often diagnosed retrospectively once a woman has had a late miscarriage or preterm labour. This may be acquired as a result of previous surgery or following childbirth. It classically presents as silent painless dilatation of the cervix and rupture of the membranes (breaking of waters) in mid-pregnancy.

Cervical weakness may be detected by transvaginal ultrasound in the early or mid-trimester. Once detected, cervical cerclage has been the mainstay of treatment. However, two randomised controlled trials did not report any significant improvement in perinatal survival from ultrasound-indicated cervical cerclage.[7,8] A small decrease in preterm birth and delivery of very low birthweight infants was reported in the 1993 Medical Research Council/RCOG trial of elective cervical cerclage. However, this did not translate into any significant improvement in perinatal survival.[9]

Women thought to benefit from cerclage are those who have had silent cervical dilatation resulting in a severe preterm birth or late pregnancy loss, congenital disorders such as diethylstilboestrol (DES) exposure, cervical trauma secondary to repeated surgical terminations, large loop excision, cold knife conisation and trachelectomy.

Vaginal cerclage (Figure 3.1) remains the preferred technique and transabdominal cerclage is only advocated in selected women with previous failed transvaginal cerclage or a very short cervix. An alternative to cerclage is transvaginal scan monitoring of the cervix and rescue cerclage when there is shortening and funnelling of the cervix. The evidence in favour of this however remains conflicting.

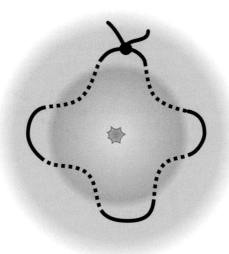

Figure 3.1 Cervical suture (published in *Clinical Obstetrics and Gynaecology*, 2nd ed., Magowan BA, Owen P, Drife J, 'Miscarriage' p. 97–102. Copyright Elsevier 2009.)[10]

ENDOCRINE FACTORS

Although maternal endocrine conditions such as diabetes mellitus and thyroid disease have been associated with miscarriage, the prevalence of these conditions among women suffering recurrent miscarriage is similar to that in the general population.[3,10] Thus, there is no evidence for undertaking routine screening for diabetes and thyroid disease with oral glucose tolerance and thyroid function tests in asymptomatic women presenting with recurrent miscarriage.[1]

Although there have been studies proving the beneficial effect of progesterone supplementation in pregnancy to prevent a miscarriage, this has not been endorsed widely and the use of progesterone to prevent miscarriage still remains in the context of research trials. A large multicentre randomised controlled study (PROMISE study) to look at the effect of progesterone supplementation in the first trimester of pregnancy in women with a history of unexplained recurrent miscarriages is currently in progress. It is hoped that this trial will provide the required evidence for recommendations in this area. The intervention arm of this study will involve the administration of 400 mg of vaginal progesterone as pessaries twice daily, started soon after confirmation of pregnancy but before 6 weeks of gestation and continued to 12 weeks of gestation. The primary outcome would be to compare the live births beyond 24 weeks in the study population.[11]

Although the prevalence of ultrasound-detected polycystic ovaries is significantly higher among women with recurrent miscarriage (41%) when compared with the general population (22%), this in itself does not predict an increased risk of future pregnancy loss among ovulatory women with a history of recurrent miscarriage following spontaneous conception.[12] Although a higher rate of miscarriage has been reported among women with polycystic ovary syndrome and known insulin resistance undergoing ovulation induction compared with those who are not insulin resistant, treatment with insulin sensitising agents such as metformin has not been proven to improve the pregnancy outcome. In women with history of recurrent miscarriage, an elevated free androgen index seems to be a prognostic factor for subsequent miscarriage.[1]

Where persistently raised levels of follicle-stimulating hormone is noted in women suffering recurrent miscarriage, they should be investigated promptly to identify possible premature ovarian failure and counselled appropriately.[3]

THROMBOPHILIA AND INHERITED THROMBOPHILIC DEFECTS

Antiphospholipid antibodies are present in 15% of women with recurrent miscarriage.[13] The main type of antiphospholipid antibodies are lupus anticoagulant, anticardiolipin antibody and anti-B2 glycoprotein-I antibodies. The association between antiphospholipid antibodies and adverse pregnancy outcomes such as recurrent miscarriage is referred to as antiphospholipid syndrome. Antiphospholipid antibodies tend to cause adverse pregnancy outcome through various mechanisms, including the inhibition of trophoblastic function and differentiation and, in later pregnancy, thrombosis of the uteroplacental vasculature.[1]

To establish a diagnosis of antiphospholipid syndrome, there should be two positive tests at least 12 weeks apart for either lupus anticoagulant or anticardiolipin antibodies of immunoglobulin G and/or M in a medium or high titre (over 40 g/l or ml/l or above the 99th percentile).[1] One positive result alone may be caused by viral or other infections.

In women with a history of recurrent miscarriage associated with antiphospholipid antibodies, treatment with low-dose aspirin and heparin in a subsequent pregnancy is found to improve future live birth rates.[1] Despite treatment, these pregnancies still remain at high risk of complications, including miscarriage, pre-eclampsia, fetal growth restriction and preterm birth, and should be managed as high-risk pregnancies requiring careful monitoring.[1]

Inherited thrombophilic defects include activated protein C resistance, most commonly factor V leiden (FVL) gene mutation, deficiencies of protein C/S and anti-thrombin III, hyperhomocystinaemia and prothrombin gene mutation have been associated with late pregnancy losses and this is thought to be as a result of thrombosis of uteroplacental circulation. Some studies have suggested that treatment with low molecular weight heparin may improve the live birth rate for these women. Although not supported by randomised trials, it is recommended that routine screening for FVL may be justified and offering thromboprophylaxis for those with FVL mutation and evidence of placental thrombosis may be of some benefit.[1]

ALLOIMMUNE FACTORS

There is no convincing evidence to suggest parental human leucocyte antigen (HLA) incompatibility or lack of maternal leucocytotoxic antibodies as contributory factors for recurrent miscarriage and so routine tests for HLA type and anti-paternal cytotoxic antibodies are not recommended.[1]

Natural killer (NK) cells found in peripheral blood and within uterine decidua has been associated with recurrent miscarriage. Researchers have postulated that raised levels of peripheral NK cell cytotoxicity is associated with recurrent miscarriage and immunosuppressive treatment with steroids may help improve pregnancy outcomes in these women.[14,15] However, based on current evidence, measurement of peripheral blood NK cells and endometrial biopsy for uterine NK cells is confined to research studies only.

INFECTION

In women with a previous history of second-trimester miscarriage or spontaneous preterm labour, screening for and treatment of bacterial vaginosis in early pregnancy may reduce the risk of recurrent late loss and preterm birth.[1] However, there is no evidence to support screening for toxoplasmosis, other (congenital syphilis and viruses), rubella, cytomegalovirus and herpes simplex virus (TORCH).[1]

Investigations

Table 3.1 shows the causes of recurrent miscarriage and suggested investigations. While the vast majority of women suffering recurrent miscarriage have no identifiable aetiology and can be classed as idiopathic, a battery of investigations can be undertaken to detect any treatable causative factor(s).

Table 3.1 Causes of recurrent miscarriage and suggested investigations

Cause	Investigations
Idiopathic	Reassurance, ultrasound scan
Genetic factors	Cytogenetic analysis of products of conception of the third and subsequent miscarriages. If this reports unbalanced structural chromosomal abnormality then undertake peripheral blood karyotyping of both partners
Anatomical factors	Pelvic ultrasound scan, including scan for cervical length during pregnancy in suspected cases of cervical weakness
Antiphospholipid syndrome	Immunoglobulin G and M anticardiolipin antibodies Lupus anticoagulant
Inherited thrombophilia defects (for second-trimester miscarriage)	Factor V Leiden mutation Factor II prothrombin gene mutation Protein C/S levels Activated protein C resistance
Hormonal factors	Early follicular phase follicle-stimulating hormone

CYTOGENETIC INVESTIGATIONS

RCOG guidelines on recurrent miscarriage suggest undertaking cytogenetic analysis of the products of conception from the third and subsequent miscarriages and to consider parental karyotyping only if the cytogenetic analysis shows an unbalanced structural chromosomal abnormality.[1] Information on karyotyping is helpful when counselling couples regarding the future pregnancy outcome.

ANATOMICAL CAUSES

Ultrasound scanning, particularly three-dimensional ultrasound, has proved to be a valuable non-invasive tool in the outpatient setting for the detection of uterine malformations in women with recurrent miscarriage.[16] In a large study comparing ultrasound morphology in women with and without recurrent miscarriage, Salim et al. found no significant difference in the prevalence of various uterine malformations between the two groups. However, for both arcuate and subseptate uteruses, the size of fundal distortion was found to be higher and the length of the remaining uterine cavity shorter in groups of women with recurrent miscarriage.[17] In addition to ultrasound scanning, in some cases hysteroscopy, laparoscopy and hysterosalpingography may help to establish the correct diagnosis.

COAGULATION DISORDERS

Screening for inherited thrombophilia defects by testing for FVL mutation, factor II prothrombin gene mutation, protein C and S levels and activated protein C resistance is deemed to be of value in women experiencing second-trimester miscarriage.

Acquired maternal thrombophilia is a well recognised cause of recurrent miscarriage and it is advisable to offer all women with recurrent first-trimester miscarriage and second-trimester miscarriage testing for antiphospholipid antibodies (lupus anticoagulant and anticardiolipin antibodies). Inter-laboratory variations and lack of standardisation of tests in the detection of antiphospholipid antibodies are well recognised issues in this area.[1]

HORMONAL INVESTIGATIONS

There is insufficient evidence to recommend routine hormonal investigations in the form of thyroid function tests, haemoglobin A1C estimation, luteinising hormone, androgen and prolactin levels in women with recurrent miscarriage. However, early follicular-phase follicle-stimulating hormone levels may be helpful in assessing a woman's ovarian function, as higher day 2/3 follicle-stimulating hormone levels are associated with lower conception rates.

Management

Management of recurrent pregnancy losses can be challenging for both the couple and clinicians and should be dictated by the results of the investigations. It may involve referral to a specialist recurrent miscarriage clinic. For the vast majority of couples there will be no identifiable cause to account for these consecutive pregnancy losses (unexplained recurrent miscarriage) and this can be extremely distressing. These women can be reassured that the prognosis for a successful future pregnancy with supportive care alone, without any pharmacological intervention, is in the region of 75%.[1] The main determinants of future pregnancy outcome are maternal age and the number of miscarriages the woman has suffered.[19] Advanced paternal age has also been identified as a risk factor for miscarriage.[1] The predicted probability of successful future pregnancy based on a woman's age and previous miscarriage history is shown in Table 3.2.[18]

Another common concern for these women is deciding the optimal timing for the next pregnancy. While some clinicians suggest delaying conception after miscarriage for a few months, the evidence on the relationship between inter-pregnancy interval and pregnancy

Table 3.2	Predicted probability (%) of a successful pregnancy by age and previous miscarriage history[18]			
Age (years)	Number of previous miscarriages (95% confidence interval)			
	2 miscarriages	3 miscarriages	4 miscarriages	5 miscarriages
20	92 (86–98)	90 (83–97)	88 (79–96)	85 (74–96)
25	89 (82–95)	86 (79–93)	82 (75–91)	79 (68–90)
30	84 (77–90)	80 (74–86)	76 (69–83)	71 (61–81)
35	77 (69–85)	73 (66–80)	68 (60–75)	62 (51–74)
40	69 (57–82)	64 (52–76)	58 (45–71)	52 (37–67)
45	60 (41–70)	54 (35–72)	48 (29–67)	42 (22–62)

outcomes is too limited to be able to provide any clear guidance. World Health Organization guidelines recommend waiting 6 months before trying to conceive again after a miscarriage.[20] However, a large retrospective study from Scotland looking at the effect of inter-pregnancy interval on outcome of pregnancy after miscarriage concluded that women who conceive within 6 months of a miscarriage have a better reproductive outcome and lower rate of pregnancy-related complications in a subsequent pregnancy.[21]

Key points

- Recurrent miscarriage affects around 1% of fertile couples.
- The risk of recurrent miscarriage increases with increasing maternal age and number of miscarriages.
- The cause of recurrent miscarriage remains unexplained in the majority of couples.
- Women suffering from recurrent miscarriage should be cared for by experts in the field and are best managed in the setting of a dedicated recurrent miscarriage clinic.
- Provision of supportive care and reassurance with ultrasound remains the most favourable intervention.

References

1. Royal College of Obstetricians and Gynaecologists. *The Investigation and Treatment of Couples with Recurrent Miscarriage*. Green-top Guideline No. 17. London: RCOG; 2011 [www.rcog.org.uk/womens-health/clinical-guidance/investigation-and-treatment-couples-recurrent-miscarriage-green-top-].
2. de Braekeleer M, Dao TN. Cytogenetic studies in couples experiencing repeated pregnancy losses. *Hum Reprod* 1990;5:519–28.
3. Clifford K, Rai R, Watson H, Regan L. An informative protocol for the investigation of recurrent miscarriage: preliminary experience of 500 consecutive cases. *Hum Reprod* 1994;9:1328–32.
4. Regan L, Rai R, Backos M, El Gaddal S. Recurrent miscarriage and parental karyotype abnormalities: prevalence and future pregnancy outcome. *Hum Reprod* 2001;16:177–8.
5. Ogilvie CM, Braude P, Scriven PN. Successful pregnancy outcomes after preimplantation genetic diagnosis (PGD) for carriers of chromosome translocations. *Hum Fertil (Camb)* 2001;4:168–71.
6. Grimbizis GF, Camus M, Tarlatzis BC, Bontis JN, Devroey P. Clinical implications of uterine malformations and hysteroscopic treatment results. *Hum Reprod Update* 2001;7:161–74.
7. Althuisius SM, Dekker GA, van Geijn HP, Bekedam DJ, Hummel P. Cervical incompetence prevention randomized cerclage trial (CIPRACT): study design and preliminary results. *Am J Obstet Gynecol* 2000;183:823–9.
8. Rust OA, Atlas RO, Jones KJ, Benham BN, Balducci J. A randomized trial of cerclage versus no cerclage among patients with ultrasonographically detected second-trimester preterm dilatation of the internal os. *Am J Obstet Gynecol* 2000;183:830–5.

9.   Medical Research Council; RCOG Working Party on Cervical Cerclage. Final Report of the Medical Research Council/Royal College of Obstetricians and Gynaecologists Multicentre Randomised Trial of Cervical Cerclage. *Br J Obstet Gynaecol* 1993;100:516–23.

10. Owen P. Miscarriage. In: Magowan BA, Owen P, Drife J. *Clinical Obstetrics and Gynaecology*. 2nd ed. London: Saunders; 2009. p. 97–102.

11. Li TC, Spuijbroek MD, Tuckerman E, Anstie B, Loxley M, Laird S. Endocrinological and endometrial factors in recurrent miscarriage. *BJOG* 2000;107:1471–9.

12. Coomaraswamy A, Truchanowicz EG, Rai R. Does first trimester progesterone prophylaxis increase the live birth rate in women with unexplained recurrent miscarriages? *BMJ* 2011;342:922–3.

13. Rai R, Backos M, Rushworth F, Regan L. Polycystic ovaries and recurrent miscarriage: a reappraisal. *Hum Reprod* 2000;15:612–15.

14. Rai RS, Regan L, Clifford K, Pickering W, Dave M, Mackie I, et al. Antiphospholipid antibodies and beta 2-glycoprotein-I in 500 women with recurrent miscarriage: results of a comprehensive screening approach. *Hum Reprod* 1995;10:2001–5.

15. Farquharson RG, Stephenson MD. *Early Pregnancy*. Cambridge: Cambridge University Press; 2010. p. 59–65.

16. Quenby S, Kalumbi C, Bates M, Farquharson R, Vince G. Prednisolone reduces preconceptual natural killer cells in women with recurrent miscarriage. *Fertil Steril* 2005;84:980–4.

17. Salim R, Woelfer B, Backos M, Regan L, Jurkovic D. Reproducibility of three-dimensional ultrasound diagnosis of congenital uterine anomalies. *Ultrasound Obstet Gynecol* 2003;21:578–82.

18. Salim R, Regan L, Woelfer B, Backos M, Jurkovic D. A comparative study of the morphology of congenital uterine anomalies in women with and without a history of recurrent first trimester miscarriage. *Hum Reprod* 2003;18:162–6.

19. Brigham S, Conlon C, Farquharson RG. A longitudinal study of pregnancy outcome following idiopathic recurrent miscarriage. *Hum Reprod* 1999;14:2868–71.

20. World Health Organization. Report of a WHO Technical Consultation on Birth Spacing. Geneva, Switzerland 13–15 June 2005. Geneva: WHO; 2007 [http://www.who.int/reproductivehealth/publications/family_planning/WHO_RHR_07_1/en/].

21. Love ER, Bhattacharya S, Smith NC, Bhattacharya S. Effect of interpregnancy interval on outcomes of pregnancy after miscarriage: retrospective analysis of hospital episode statistics in Scotland. *BMJ* 2010;341:c3967.

4   Ectopic pregnancy

Ectopic pregnancy is pregnancy located outside the uterine cavity. This condition occurs in approximately 1/90 pregnancies (just over 1%) in the UK. Evidence suggests that the incidence of ectopic pregnancies has been rising. While this increase is for the most part aided by better diagnostic techniques, early diagnosis also plays a role by identifying ectopic pregnancies that may otherwise have spontaneously resolved. Although it rarely presents as a life-threatening emergency in the UK, ectopic pregnancy still remains the leading cause of maternal death in the first trimester and contributed to ten maternal deaths in the triennium 2003–2005.[1] Box 4.1 lists the aetiology and predisposing factors for ectopic pregnancy.

BOX 4.1 AETIOLOGY AND PREDISPOSING FACTORS FOR ECTOPIC PREGNANCY

- Previous ectopic pregnancy
- Past or present pelvic inflammatory disease: the most common cause being infection with *Chlamydia trachomatis*
- Pregnancy with intrauterine contraceptive device in place
- Pregnancy resulting from failure of progestogen-only pill
- Previous pelvic surgery, including caesarean section and tubal surgery (including sterilisation, appendicectomy)
- Pregnancy following assisted conception techniques
- Pregnancy in women over 40 years of age
- Pregnancy in women who smoke

Presentation

The large majority (95%) of ectopic pregnancies occur in the fallopian tube, the ampullary part of the tube being the most common implantation site (70%) followed by isthmic (12%) and fimbrial (11.1%) locations. However, ectopic pregnancies can occur in other

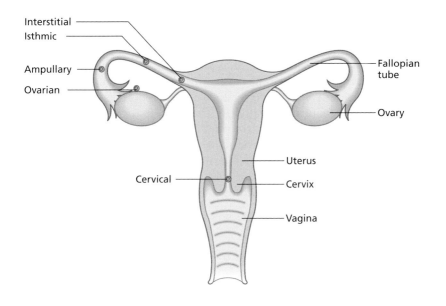

Interstitial

Isthmic

Ampullary

Ovarian

Fallopian tube

Ovary

Uterus

Cervical

Cervix

Vagina

Figure 4.1 Sites of ectopic pregnancy (reproduced with permission from *British Medical Journal* 320 (7239), Tay JI, Moore J, Walker JJ, Ectopic pregnancy. Copyright © 2000, British Medical Journal Publishing Group)

locations such as the ovary, cervix and abdominal cavity. Non-tubal ectopic pregnancies, although infrequent, tend to present a diagnostic dilemma and are often associated with more serious consequences to the woman than tubal ectopic pregnancies.[2] Cornual or interstitial pregnancies account for approximately 1–6% of ectopic pregnancies and cervical pregnancies account for less than 1% of ectopic pregnancies. Ovarian pregnancies account for 0.5–3.0% of all ectopic pregnancies and caesarean ectopics, whereby the pregnancy is located in the caesarean scar, can be seen in up to 6% of all ectopic pregnancies in women with previous caesarean sections. Combined intrauterine and extrauterine pregnancy (heterotopic pregnancy) is rarely encountered, with an incidence of approximately 1/40 000 natural pregnancies and 1/1000 pregnancies following in vitro fertilisation. Figure 4.1 shows locations of ectopic pregnancies.

Clinical presentation in ectopic pregnancy is variable, ranging from asymptomatic to signs of peritonism and collapse. The majority of women with symptoms of ectopic pregnancy are referred to hospital and seen in the early pregnancy assessment unit (EPAU). A detailed history should be elicited, looking for risk factors for ectopic pregnancy, as these may be noted in almost 25–50% of women.[3] The old axiom that every woman with abdominal pain with or without bleeding in early pregnancy has an ectopic pregnancy unless proven otherwise still remains pertinent today.[3] The 2003–2005 report on Confidential Enquiries into Maternal Deaths in the United Kingdom specifically recommends practitioners to consider the possibility of ectopic pregnancy in all women of reproductive age group who present with diarrhoea and vomiting and/or fainting to avoid the pitfall of missing this potentially serious condition.[1] Women commonly present with a combination of the symptoms shown in Box 4.2.[4–7]

Diagnosis

Ultrasonography and estimation of serum beta hCG (βhCG) are the two key tools for assessment of women presenting with pain with or without bleeding in early pregnancy. Early diagnosis of ectopic pregnancy is achieved by a high index of suspicion, transvaginal ultrasonography and quantitative serum βhCG estimation. A transvaginal ultrasound scan can reveal intrauterine pregnancies at an earlier stage and detect a greater proportion of ectopic pregnancies. The higher specificity (over 98%) of transvaginal ultrasonography compared with the transabdominal route (60–80%) in diagnosing an ectopic pregnancy by detection of an adnexal mass makes the former the investigation of choice.[2]

Visualisation of a yolk sac or fetal pole with gestation sac inside the uterus is necessary to exclude ectopic pregnancy. An intrauterine pregnancy is usually detectable on transabdominal ultrasound at a βhCG level greater than 6500 iu/litre and on transvaginal ultrasound when serum βhCG levels exceed 1500 iu/litre (discriminatory zone).[8] An ectopic pregnancy is highly likely if a scan detects an adnexal mass in the absence of an intrauterine pregnancy when serum βhCG levels are more than 1500 iu/litre (Figure 4.2). If, however, the serum βhCG level is below 1500 iu/litre and transvaginal ultrasound fails to reveal an intrauterine or ectopic pregnancy, it is advisable to repeat these examinations every 48–72 hours until a definitive diagnosis is established.

The value of a single reading of serum βhCG (discriminatory zone) in differentiating ectopic pregnancy from intrauterine pregnancy, however, has been challenged in a 2011 study.[9] Serum βhCG levels usually double every 2–3 days and non-doubling has been deemed highly suggestive of nonviable pregnancies, including ectopic and

BOX 4.2 DIAGNOSIS OF ECTOPIC PREGNANCY

Clinical: Symptoms of ectopic pregnancy include:

- History of amenorrhea: usually 6–8 weeks although may present at any stage
- Pelvic pain and/or abnormal bleeding in the first trimester. Bleeding occurs as a result of shedding of decidua from uterine cavity and is generally light
- Shoulder tip pain or discomfort as a result of diaphragmatic irritation from intraperitoneal bleeding
- Dizziness or spells of fainting
- Other evidence of blood in the peritoneal cavity causing peritoneal irritation resulting in pain on defecation or diarrhoea

Bio-chemical:

- Positive pregnancy test (urine or serum)

On transvaginal sonography:

- No evidence of intrauterine gestational sac
- Positive visualisation of an extrauterine pregnancy: tubal ectopic pregnancy may be diagnosed when an adnexal mass is noted separate to the ovary (Figure 4.2). The mass may be an inhomogenous adnexal mass or an empty extrauterine sac with a hyperechoic ring or a yolk sac with or without fetal pole with or without cardiac activity in an extrauterine sac.[4,5,6] An adnexal mass will not be found in 15–35% of women with an ectopic pregnancy
- Free fluid in the pouch of Douglas may suggest haemoperitoneum
- Collection of fluid within the endometrial cavity often referred to as a 'pseudosac'. This should, however, be distinguished from a true intrauterine sac, which is seen as an eccentrically placed hyperechoic ring within the endometrial cavity (Table 4.1)[7]

intrauterine pregnancies that are destined to miscarry. However, it is increasingly recognised that patterns of serum βhCG secretion in ectopic pregnancies may not be greatly different from those seen in normal and abnormal intrauterine pregnancies, making it more diffi-cult to establish a definitive diagnosis of the exact location of pregnancy based on serum βhCG values.[10]

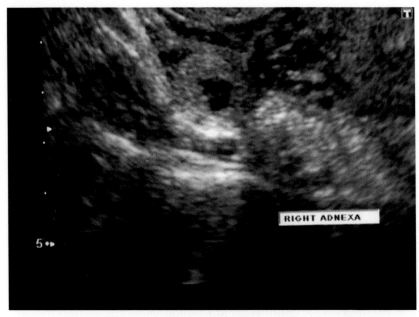

Figure 4.2 Right-sided adnexal mass later confirmed as tubal pregnancy on laparoscopy

An estimation of serum progesterone levels may be helpful in reaching a diagnosis in some cases. The level of serum progesterone is noted to be higher in women with viable intrauterine pregnancy than those with non-viable intrauterine or ectopic pregnancy. However, the progesterone levels are found to be low in both failing intrauterine or ectopic pregnancies, making it difficult to differentiate between the two.[8]

Table 4.1 Differential diagnosis between early intrauterine gestational sac and pseudosac[11]

	Early gestational sac	Pseudosac
Location	Below the midline echo buried into the endometrium	Along the cavity line between endometrial layers
Shape	Steady, usually round	May change during scan, usually ovoid
Borders	Double ring	Single layer
Colour flow pattern	High peripheral flow	Avascuar

Although single measurements of hormones are not of value on their own, follow-up of these values in combination with ultrasonography helps to reach a diagnosis in the majority of women. Transvaginal ultrasound offers an accurate diagnosis for ectopic pregnancy, with a sensitivity as high as 87–99% and specificity of 94–99%.[12,13] An overall sensitivity of 98.3% with a specificity of 99.9%, a positive predictive value of 97.5% and a negative predictive value of 100% has been quoted by Kirk et al. in their study looking at diagnostic effectiveness of the initial transvaginal ultrasound scan in detecting ectopic pregnancy within an EPAU setting.[12] Positive visualisation of an ectopic pregnancy on ultrasound scan is diagnostic, while absence of intrauterine or extrauterine pregnancy in the presence of a positive pregnancy test should be classed as 'pregnancy of unknown location' and managed accordingly. It is vital to carefully follow up these women with serum βhCG tests and/or scans until the final outcome is established, as a significant proportion of women with pregnancies of unknown location (7–20%) will subsequently be diagnosed with ectopic pregnancy.[6] Measurement of endometrial thickness in the absence of intrauterine pregnancy has not been found to be of help in reaching a diagnosis.[13]

Dilatation and curettage is now rarely advisable for diagnostic purposes. However, in cases where evacuation of retained products of conception has been performed with a diagnosis of miscarriage, one must check the histology with urgent recall for further investigations to rule out ectopic pregnancy if histology reveals decidua only in the absence of chorionic villi: Arias–Stella reaction.[3] Laparoscopy remains the gold standard for diagnosis of extrauterine pregnancy with a false negative result in up to 4–5% of cases (Figure 4.3).

Management

The management of ectopic pregnancy has changed significantly over the years and has shifted from a surgical approach by laparotomy to either expectant or medical or minimally invasive laparoscopic surgery. Management should always be tailored to the clinical condition of the patient and her future fertility demands. Figure 4.4 provides an algorithm for the management of ectopic pregnancy.

SURGICAL MANAGEMENT

Women who are haemodynamically unstable or who choose to have surgical treatment or those who are not suitable for medical treatment should be offered surgical management.

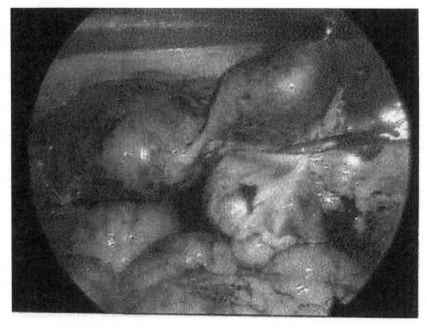

Figure 4.3 Right-sided tubal ectopic pregnancy at laparoscopy

Laparotomy or laparoscopy?

Randomised controlled trials comparing laparotomy with laparoscopy have reported that the laparoscopic approach was associated with significantly less blood loss, lower analgesia requirements, shorter hospital stay and quicker postoperative recovery time.[14] The subsequent intrauterine pregnancy rate was 70% after laparoscopic surgery compared with 55% after laparotomy. The recurrent ectopic pregnancy rate was also lower with laparoscopic treatment at 5% compared with 16.6% with laparotomy. The incidence of adhesion formation is also noted to be higher among women undergoing laparotomy.[15]

The laparoscopic approach has now become the norm for women who are haemodynamically stable. In some centres this is the preferred approach even in the presence of haemoperitoneum but management would depend on the expertise available locally. It is recommended that haemostasis is secured immediately after laparoscope insertion by anteflexing the uterus and identifying the fallopian tube. The evacuation of haemoperitoneum can be safely performed after controlling the bleeding.[16]

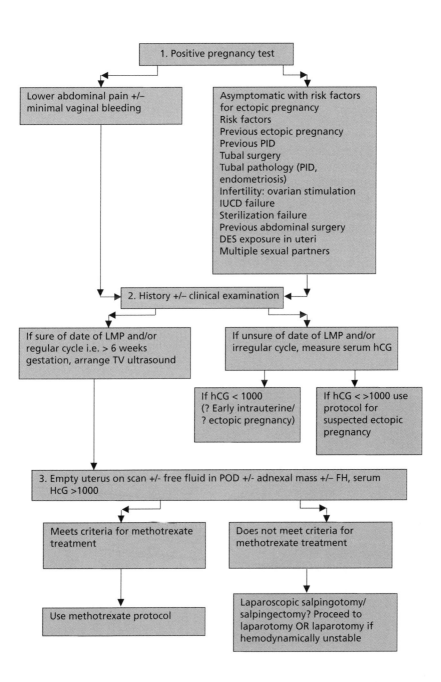

Figure 4.4 Management algorithm for ectopic pregnancy (adapted from Mascarenhas LJ, 'Problems in early pregnancy' in *Obstetrics and Gynaecology: An evidence-based text for MRCOG*, Wesley DM and Baker PN, p. 606–15)[3]

If the woman is not haemodynamically stable, the most expedient method of surgical management should be chosen; in most cases this will be a laparotomy.

Salpingectomy or salpingostomy?

Salpingectomy (total) (Figure 4.5) is to be preferred to salpingotomy when the contralateral tube is healthy, as it is associated with lower rates of persistent trophoblast and subsequent repeat ectopic pregnancy while having similar subsequent intrauterine pregnancy rates (approximately 45%).[14] Linear salpingotomy should be considered as the primary treatment for unruptured tubal pregnancy if the woman has contralateral tubal disease and desires future fertility. This is performed by making a one-centimetre incision on the anti-mesosalpinx using monopolar needle cautery and the products of conception are flushed out using a suction irrigator. Any bleeding can be controlled by using fine-tip cautery or pressure. The tubal opening is usually left open to heal by secondary intention.[17] Women undergoing salpingotomy require regular follow up with quantitative hCG estimation. It is advisable to undertake a day 3 βhCG and day 7 βhCG estimation

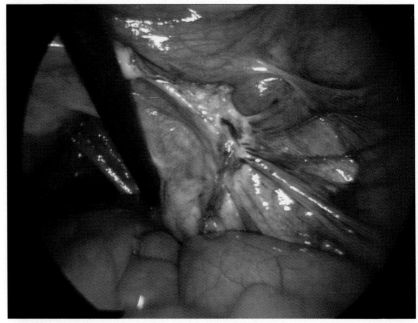

Figure 4.5 Laparoscopic view after salpingectomy for tubal ectopic pregnancy

post-salpingotomy. If βhCG plateaus or rises, an ultrasound scan should be repeated and medical treatment with methotrexate or repeat surgery should be considered. Where a suboptimal fall in βhCG precedes a negative laparoscopy, expectant management may be considered appropriate. An overall rate of 15.4% is quoted for recurrent ectopic pregnancy after linear salpingotomy.[18]

MEDICAL MANAGEMENT

Single-dose methotrexate is the most widely accepted medical treatment for ectopic pregnancy. Medical treatment should be offered to properly selected patients (Box 4.3) and should be based on strict protocols, with women having immediate access to inpatient facilities if complications occur. Methotrexate is a folic acid antagonist which prevents the growth of rapidly dividing cells by interfering with DNA synthesis. Administered as a single dose of 50 mg/m^2 body surface area, a resorption rate of 92% (success rates) and subsequent intrauterine pregnancy rates of 58% with a recurrent ectopic rate of 9% has been

---

BOX 4.3 SELECTION OF WOMEN SUITABLE FOR MEDICAL TREATMENT

Medical treatment is most suitable for women who:

- are haemodynamically stable with no signs of active intra-abdominal bleeding
- have βhCG less than 5000 miu/litre^2
- have no fetal heart activity on ultrasound, an unruptured ectopic mass size less than 3.5 cm
- will be compliant with regular follow ups
- agree to use reliable contraceptive for at least 3 months following treatment
- desire future fertility
- have no pre-existing severe medical condition or disorder
- have no evidence of liver, renal or bone marrow impairment
- have no known contraindications to methotrexate
- are not currently taking nonsteroidal anti-inflammatory drugs, diuretics, penicillin or tetracycline group drugs (this is not so critical for the single-dose methotrexate regimen)
- do not have a coexisting intrauterine pregnancy
- are not breastfeeding.

reported.[19] Morlock et al., in a meta-analysis, revealed similar success rates for methotrexate treatment and laparoscopic salpingostomy (72–100%).[20] Approximately 14% of women require a second dose of methotrexate, while 7% may experience tubal rupture and require surgery. Seventy-five percent of women experience abdominal pain as a result of tubal miscarriage or formation of hematoma with tubal distension following administration of methotrexate and it may be difficult at times to differentiate between tubal miscarriage and tubal rupture. The clinical scan findings should help to dictate the management. Most women respond to conservative management and may need a short period of hospitalisation for close observation. Some women may experience minor adverse effects such as stomatitis or alopecia but these are rare with one or two doses.

Women undergoing this form of treatment should be advised of the possibility of experiencing abdominal pain and provided with a written information leaflet informing them of the need to seek medical attention in such situations. Women should be advised to avoid consuming alcohol, vitamins, aspirin, nonsteroidal anti-inflammatory drugs and excessive exposure to sun (risk of photosensitive skin reaction) in the immediate post treatment period.

A high serum hCG level is found to be the most important prognostic factor of the failure of methotrexate treatment.[21] Gazvani et al. compared methotrexate alone with a combination of mifepristone (anti-prostaglandin) and methotrexate and noted the resolution time to be shorter with less likelihood of needing a second dose of methotrexate or laparotomy in the combination arm.[22] Box 4.4 gives a protocol for treatment with methotrexate.

The psychological impact of early pregnancy loss may seriously affect women and their partners. A study looking at the impact of treatment on women's health-related quality of life showed a marginally higher negative impact following medical treatment when compared with surgical treatment, citing a possible risk of tubal rupture and the need for prolonged follow-up as the likely causes of distress.[23] Women should be appropriately counselled and informed consent sought before recommending any treatment.

An economic comparison of the two modalities by Mol et al. from the Netherlands in 1999 found methotrexate treatment to be less costly when the initial serum βhCG was less than 1500 miu/ml and comparatively more expensive when the initial hCG was greater than 3000 miu/ml.[24]

BOX 4.4 PROTOCOL FOR TREATMENT WITH METHOTREXATE

SELECTION:

- Select women suitable for medical treatment carefully according to agreed criteria or local policy and ensure appropriate counselling.
- Women should be provided with written information and seeking a written consent is considered good practice.

Day 1   Methotrexate given. Check full blood count (FBC), urea and electrolytes (U&E), blood group and antibody

Day 4   Routine observations and βhCG estimation. Serum hCG level on day 4 may be slightly higher than pretreatment levels

Day 7   Routine observations and FBC, βhCG, liver function tests (LFTs), U&E

Day 14   FBC, βhCG

FOLLOW-UP:

Weekly follow-up in EPAU until βhCG is less than 25 iu/litre. βhCG can take up to 4 weeks or more to fall. If βhCG does not fall by greater than 15% between days 4 and 7 or becomes static after an initial fall, a second dose of methotrexate can be given (required in around 15% of cases, administered in the opposite gluteal region). If a second dose is administered, follow-up arrangements should be made for measurement of βhCG, FBC, LFTs and U&E.

EXPECTANT MANAGEMENT

An early diagnosis of ectopic pregnancy allows a small window of opportunity to offer expectant management to selected women. There have been two published randomised controlled trials on expectant management of ectopic pregnancy.[25,26] The first compared expectant management with local or systemic prostaglandins and expectant management was noted to be less successful than prostaglandin treatment (relative risk 0.12, 95% CI 0.02–0.81). The second trial of expectant management compared with oral methotrexate in a low dose of

2.5 mg/day for 5 days revealed similar success rates of 77% in both treatment groups (relative risk 1.0, 95% CI 0.76–1.3).

Success rates of up to 69% have been noted in one prospective study looking at conservative management.[16] However, the majority of the studies included women with pregnancy of unknown location in the expectant management group and the role of this form of management in those with a definite ectopic pregnancy remains less clear. Using a combination of serum hCG and serum progesterone level, one may be able to select this form of treatment (Table 4.2).

Table 4.2 Laboratory indices in the diagnosis of ectopic pregnancy[3]

Serum progesterone (nmol/l)	Serum βhCG (IU/l)	Prognosis	Follow-up
< 20	< 25	Reassuring	Blood/urine hCG in 7 days
20–60	> 25	High risk of ectopic	Serum hCG in 48 hours
> 60	< 1000	Low risk of ectopic	Repeat scan when hCG > 1000 IU/l
> 60	> 1000	Ectopic	Repeat scan as soon as possible ± laparoscopy

Non-tubal ectopic pregnancy

The management of non-tubal ectopic pregnancy will depend on the exact location and can be more complex. Non-tubal ectopic pregnancy is known to be associated with higher morbidity and mortality and early diagnosis provides a scope for offering the best possible treatment option in these cases.

INTERSTITIAL PREGNANCY

Interstitial pregnancy accounts for approximately 2.5% of all ectopic pregnancies. It is diagnosed on ultrasound visualisation of an interstitial line adjoining the gestational sac and the lateral aspect of the uterine cavity and continuation of the myometrial mantle around the ectopic sac.[27] Although traditionally these cases were managed by surgical resection at laparotomy, laparoscopic management and even medical treatment with local or systemic methotrexate or expectant management has been reported with good results. Expectant management is most suitable for women with low levels of hCG or falling levels of hCG. Success rates as high as 94% have been reported using a single dose of intramuscular methotrexate (50 mg/m²).[28] Occasional cases have been managed with adjunctive use of selective uterine artery embolisation together with methotrexate to help reduce the bleeding, although the safety of this technique with regard to future pregnancies remains doubtful.[29]

CORNUAL PREGNANCY

Although the terms 'cornual' and 'interstitial' pregnancy have been used interchangeably, a true cornual pregnancy is one which is implanted in the rudimentary horn of a unicornuate uterus and is a very rare phenomenon.[30] Ultrasound criteria for diagnosing corneal pregnancy are visualisation of a gestational sac separate from the uterus surrounded by myometrium and a single interstitial portion of the fallopian tube in the main uterine body together with a vascular connection between the gestational sac and the unicornuate uterus. These cases are best managed by laparoscopic or open excision of the rudimentary horn.

CAESAREAN-SCAR PREGNANCY

Caesarean-scar pregnancy, although a relatively rare entity, is thought to be of significance because of the rise in caesarean sections in developed countries. Previous caesarean section, myomectomy, dilatation and curettage and manual removal of an adherent placenta have all been known to increase the risk of pregnancy implanting in the caesarean scar.[30] Ultrasound aided by Doppler, hysteroscopy and magnetic resonance imaging could be used to reach this diagnosis. Jurkovic et al. have described the criteria for establishing the diagnosis of caesarean scar pregnancy:

- empty uterine cavity
- gestational sac located at the level of internal os covering the visible or presumed site of previous lower segment caesarean scar
- presence of trophoblast on Doppler
- negative 'sliding organs sign'.[31]

Once diagnosed, the mode of treatment depends on the clinical condition of the patient. While laparotomy and hysterectomy seem to be the most appropriate treatment in those with significant haemoperitoneum, there have been few case reports of successful treatment with expectant or medical treatment with methotrexate. Expectant management alone, however, carries a significant risk of emergency surgery and is not considered appropriate.[30] Local injection of 25 mg methotrexate transvaginally into the pregnancy performed under ultrasound guidance has a reported 70–80% success rate.[31] Successful treatment with systemic methotrexate in combination with dilatation and evacuation has also been reported.[32] Jurkovic et al. reported in 2003 on the largest series of 18 cases of caesarean scar pregnancy and using suction curettage under ultrasound guidance followed by balloon tamponade with Foley's catheter in the presence of significant bleeding.[31] Other case studies have reported the use of uterine artery embolisation or even a Shirodkar cervical suture as an adjunct to surgical evacuation to minimise the blood loss.[11,33]

CERVICAL PREGNANCY

Cervical pregnancy accounts for less than 1% of ectopic pregnancies and results from implantation of the blastocyst within the endocervical mucosal lining. Predisposing factors include previous cervical instrumentation, synechiae, intrauterine contraceptive device use and anatomical cervical abnormalities.[30] On clinical examination, an enlarged, distended cervix with dilatation of external os may be noted.[34] On ultrasound, it is important to distinguish between a cervical ectopic pregnancy and an intrauterine pregnancy with relatively low implantation in the isthmic region or an intrauterine pregnancy in the process of miscarriage. Kung et al.[35] have described sonographic criteria for cervical ectopic pregnancy and these include an empty uterus with a barrel shaped cervix with gestational sac below the level of uterine arteries, absent sliding sign and colour Doppler flow around the sac.

Once confronted with a diagnosis of cervical pregnancy, conservative, medical or surgical treatment or a combination of these can be initiated, as there is no agreed consensus on the best modality of treatment. Surgical debulking or local injection with methotrexate, in addition to intramuscular methotrexate, has been used successfully. Adjunctive techniques such as uterine artery ligation or uterine artery embolisation have been tried to help control excessive blood loss but the safety of these remains questionable.

OVARIAN PREGNANCY

Ovarian pregnancy contributes nearly 3% of all ectopic pregnancies. Previous pelvic inflammatory disease, endometriosis, intrauterine contraceptive device use and assisted reproductive techniques have been quoted as risk factors. Spielberg, in 1878, first described the criteria for diagnosis of ovarian pregnancy on histological examination and these included:

- an entirely normal fallopian tube
- pregnancy sac located in the ovary
- ovary and gestational sac connected to the ovarian ligament
- placental tissue in the ovarian cortex.[30]

However, the diagnosis today would usually be made on ultrasound. Ovarian pregnancy usually appears as a cyst with a wide echogenic outside ring within or on the ovary. This can be mistaken for corpus luteal cyst and Doppler ultrasonography has not been shown to be particularly useful in distinguishing the two. It is therefore recommended that thick-walled ovarian cysts with an empty uterus and a serum βhCG above the discriminatory zone should be investigated to rule out ovarian ectopic pregnancy.[30] Laparoscopic removal of the ectopic pregnancy with conservation of healthy ovarian tissue and medical management with methotrexate can be used successfully in these cases.

ABDOMINAL PREGNANCY

Abdominal pregnancy contributes less than 2% of ectopic pregnancies and is extremely rare. It could be classed as primary abdominal or secondary when a tubal pregnancy has miscarried and implanted in the abdominal cavity. Gerli et al.[36] have described the diagnostic criteria on ultrasound scan as:

- absent intrauterine pregnancy
- no evidence of adnexal mass in the tube/ovary
- gestational sac surrounded by bowel loops and separated by peritoneum
- wide mobility of the pregnancy sac with probe pressure in the posterior cul-de-sac.

Surgical treatment with laparotomy or laparoscopy with or without adjuvant therapy with methotrexate has been reported for treatment of these cases.

Counselling regarding future prognosis

Women should be advised to seek medical advice early in subsequent pregnancies and recourse to early ultrasound to confirm intrauterine pregnancy, even if they are asymptomatic.

Recurrence rates of 7–10% are reported for ectopic pregnancies and this really depends on the type of surgery undertaken for treatment, apart from any underlying tubal damage.

Key points

- The estimated prevalence of ectopic pregnancy in the UK is approximately 1/90 pregnancies (just over 1%).
- Ectopic pregnancy remains an important cause of maternal morbidity and mortality.
- The possibility of ectopic pregnancy must be considered in all woman of child-bearing age presenting with symptoms of abdominal pain or bleeding or gastrointestinal symptoms.
- The combination of transvaginal scan and measurement of serum βhCG is the best method of reaching a timely diagnosis of ectopic pregnancy.
- Laparoscopic treatment is the mainstay of management of ectopic pregnancy, although selected women may be treated expectantly or with methotrexate.

References

1. Neilson J. Early pregnancy deaths. In: Lewis G, editor. The Confidential Enquiry into Maternal and Child Health (CEMACH). *Saving Mothers' Lives: Reviewing Maternal Deaths to Make Motherhood Safer 2003–2005*. The Seventh Report on Confidential Enquiries into Maternal Deaths in the United Kingdom. London: CEMACH; 2007. p. 93.
2. Jurkovic D, Wilkinson H. Diagnosis and management of ectopic pregnancy. *BMJ* 2011;342:d3397.
3. Mascarenhas LJ. Problems in early pregnancy. In: Luesley DM, Baker PN, editors. *Obstetrics and Gynaecology: An evidence-based text for MRCOG*. London: Arnold; 2004. p. 606–15.
4. Tulandi T. New protocols for ectopic pregnancy. *Contemp Obstet Gynecol* 1999;44:42–55.
5. Condous G, Okaro E, Khalid A, et al. The accuracy of transvaginal ultrasonography for the diagnosis of ectopic pregnancy prior to surgery. *Hum Reprod* 2005;20:1404–1409.
6. Kirk E, Bourne T. Diagnosis of ectopic pregnancy with ultrasound. *Best Pract Res Clin Obset Gynaecol* 2009;23:501–8.
7. Jurkovic D. Ectopic pregnancy. In: Edmonds DK, editor. *Dewhurst's Textbook of Obstetrics and Gynaecology*. 7th edition. Oxford: Wiley-Blackwell; 2007. p. 106–16.
8. Timor-Tritsch IE, Goldstein SR. *Ultrasound in Gynecology*. 2nd edition. New York: Churchill; 2006.

9. Wang R, Reynolds TA, West HH, Ravikumar D, Martinez C, McAlpine I, et al. Use of a βhCG discriminatory zone with bedside pelvic ultrasonography. *Ann Emerg Med* 2011;58:12–20.
10. Murray H, Baakdah H, Bardell T, Tulandi T. Diagnosis and treatment of ectopic pregnancy. *CMAJ* 2005;173:905–12.
11. Marchiolé P, Gorlero F, de Caro G, Podestà M, Valenzano M. Intramural pregnancy embedded in a previous caesarean section scar treated conservatively. *Ultrasound Obstet Gynecol* 2004:23:305–9.
12. Kirk E, Papgeorghiou AT, Condous G, Tan L, Bora S, Bourne T. The diagnostic effectiveness of an initial transvaginal scan in detecting ectopic pregnancy. *Hum Reprod* 2007;22:2824–8.
13. Tulandi T, Sammour A. Evidence based management of ectopic pregnancy. *Curr Opin Obstet Gynecol* 2000;12:289–92.
14. Royal College of Obstetricians and Gynaecologists. *The Management of Tubal Pregnancy*. Green-top Guideline No. 21. London: RCOG; 2004 [www.rcog.org.uk/womens-health/clinical-guidance/management-tubal-pregnancy-21-may-2004].
15. Lundorff P, Hahlin M, Källfelt B, Thorburn J, Lindblom B. Adhesion formation after laparoscopic surgery in tubal pregnancy: a randomized trial versus laparotomy. *Fertil Steril* 1991;55:911–15.
16. Tulandi T, Kabli N. Laparoscopy in patients with bleeding ectopic pregnancy. *J Obstet Gynecol Can* 2006:28:361–5.
17. Tulandi T, Guralnick M. Treatment of tubal ectopic pregnancy by salpingotomy with or without tubal suturing and salpingectomy. *Fertil Steril* 1991;55:53–5.
18. Yao M, Tulandi T. Current status of surgical and nonsurgical management of ectopic pregnancy. *Fertil Steril* 1997;67:421–33.
19. Glock JL, Johnson JV, Brumsted JR. Efficacy and safety of single dose methotrexate in the treatment of ectopic pregnancy. *Fertil Steril* 1994;62:716–21.
20. Morlock RJ, Lafata JE, Eiseenstein D. Cost effectiveness of single dose methotrexate compared with laparoscopic treatment of ectopic pregnancy. *Obstet Gynecol* 2000;95:407–12.
21. Lipscomb GH, McCord ML, Stovall TG, Huff G, Portera SG, Ling FW. Predictors of success of methotrexate treatment in women with tubal ectopic pregnancies. *N Engl J Med* 1999;341:1974–8.
22. Gazvani MR, Baruah DN, Alfirevic Z, Emery SJ. Mifepristone in combination with methotrexate for the medical treatment of tubal pregnancy; a randomized controlled trial. *Hum Reprod* 1998;13:198–90.
23. Nieuwkerk PT, Hajenius PJ, Ankum WM, Van der Veen F, Wijker W, Bossuyt PM. Systemic methotrexate therapy versus laparoscopic salpingostomy in patients with tubal pregnancy. Part 1. Impact on patients' health related quality of life. *Fertil Steril* 1998;70:511–17.
24. Mol BW, Hajenius PJ, Engelsbel S, Ankum WM, Hemrika DJ, Van der Veen F, et al. Treatment of tubal pregnancy in the Netherlands. an economic comparison of systemic methotrexate administration and laparoscopic salpingostomy. *Am J Obstet Gynecol* 1999;181:845–51.
25. Egarter C, Kiss H, Husslein P. Prostaglandin versus expectant management in early tubal pregnancy. *Prostaglandins Leukot Essen Fatty Acids* 1991;42:177–9.
26. Korhonen J, Stenman UH, Ylostalo P. Serum human chorionic dynamics during spontaneous resolution of ectopic pregnancy. *Fertil Steril* 194;61:632–6.
27. Jurkovic D, Marvelos D. Catch me if you can: ultrasound diagnosis of ectopic pregnancy. *Ultrasound Obstet Gynecol* 2007:30:1–7.
28. Jermy K, Thomas J, Doo A, Bourne T. The conservative management of interstitial pregnancy. *BJOG* 2004;111:1283–8.
29. Deruelle P, Lucot JP, Lions C, Robert Y. Management of interstitial pregnancy using selective uterine embolisation. *Obstet Gynecol* 2005;106:1165–67.
30. Chetty M, Elson J. Treating non-tubal ectopic pregnancy. *Best Pract Res Clin Obstet Gynecol* 2009;23:529–38.

31. Jurkovic D, Hillaby K, Woelfer B, Lawrence A, Salim R, Elson CJ. First trimester diagnosis and management of pregnancies implanted into the lower uterine segment caesarean scar. *Ultrasound Obstet Gynecol* 2003:21;220–7.
32. Graesslin O, Dedecker F Jr, Quereux C, Gabriel R. Conservative treatment of ectopic pregnancy in a caesarean scar. *Obstet Gynecol* 2005:105:869–71.
33. Jurkovic D, Ben-Nagi J, Offili-Yebovi D, et al. Efficacy of Shirodkar cervical suture in securing haemostasis following surgical evacuation of caesarean scar ectopic pregnancy. *Ultrasound Obstet Gynecol* 2007;30:95–100.
34. Ushakov FB, Elchalal U, Aceman PJ, Schenker JG. Cervical pregnancy: past and future. *Obstet Gynecol Surv* 1997;52:45–59.
35. Kung FT, Chang SY. Efficacy of methotrexate treatment in viable and non-viable cervical pregnancies. *Am J Obstet Gynecol* 1999;181:1438–44.
36. Gerli S, Rossetti D, Baiocchi G, Clerici G, Unfer V, Di Renzo GC. Early ultrasonographic diagnosis and laparoscopic treatment of abdominal pregnancy. *Eur J Obstet Gynecol Reprod Biol* 2004;113:103–5.

5 Trophoblastic disease

Gestational trophoblastic disease (GTD) defines a continuum of a neoplastic process that arises from the fetal chorion of the placenta (trophoblast). This group of disorders consists of diseases with a varying propensity for local invasion and metastasis. The World Health Organization (WHO) has classified GTD as two premalignant diseases consisting of complete or classical hydatidiform mole (CHM) and partial hydatidiform mole (PHM) and as three malignant disorders consisting of invasive mole, choriocarcinoma and placental site trophoblastic tumour (PSTT). The last three conditions are often collectively referred to as gestational trophoblastic neoplasia (GTN).

Epidemiology

Estimates for the incidence of various forms of GTD vary in different regions of the world. The incidence of molar pregnancy in Japan (2/1000 pregnancies) is three times greater than the reported incidence in Europe or North America (0.6–1.1/1000 pregnancies). In Taiwan, 1/125 pregnancies is molar, while in the USA the incidence is 1/1500 live births. In Ireland, the incidence of CHM and PHM has been determined to be 1/1945 and 1/695, respectively, by reviewing the pathology of all products of conception from first and second trimester terminations. GTN may develop after a molar pregnancy, a non-molar pregnancy or a live birth. Gestational choriocarcinoma occurs in approximately 1/20 000–40 000 pregnancies: approximately 50% after term pregnancies, 25% after molar pregnancies and the remainder after other gestational events. PSTT is much rarer than hydatidiform moles or gestational choriocarcinoma and can develop after any type of pregnancy.[1]

The incidence of GTD in the UK is about 1/714 live births. There is evidence of ethnic variation in the incidence of GTD in the UK, with women from Asia having a higher incidence (1/387 live births) compared with non-Asian women (1/752 live births).[2]

The varying incidence of GTD may in part result from reporting population-based versus hospital based data. The high incidence in some population can also be attributed to socioeconomic and nutritional factors. The decreasing incidence of molar pregnancy in South Korea has been attributed to a more western diet and improved standard of living. Case–control studies have shown that the rate of CHM increases with decreasing intake of dietary carotene (vitamin A precursor) and animal fat. Maternal age and reproductive history also influence the rate of molar pregnancy. Women above the age of 40 years have a 5–10-fold greater risk of having a CHM, while one in three pregnancies in women above the age of 50 years results in molar gestation. A history of prior spontaneous miscarriage and infertility also appears to increase the risk of a molar gestation.[3] There does not appear to be a consistent association between maternal age and PHM. PHM appears to be more common in women with a history of irregular menses and the use of oral contraceptives for more than 4 years, but not dietary factors.[3]

Pathology and cytogenetic features

Partial and complete hydatidiform moles are distinct disease processes with typical cytogenetic, histological and clinical features. The distinctive features of these two disorders are shown in Table 5.1.

When GTN occurs after a molar pregnancy, it may have the histological pattern of either molar tissue or choriocarcinoma. Where it occurs after a non-molar pregnancy, GTN characteristically has only the histological features of choriocarcinoma. Gestational choriocarcinoma does not contain chorionic villi but is composed of sheets of both anaplastic cyto- and syncytiotrophoblast. PSTT is an uncommon variant of choriocarcinoma and is composed almost entirely of mononuclear intermediate trophoblast. It does not contain chorionic villi. PSTTs secrete very small amounts of hCG and so a large tumour burden may be present before hCG levels are detectable. PSTTs are associated with a higher percentage of free beta-hCG which can contribute to diagnosis. Serum human placental lactogen (hPL) can also be used to monitor PSTT.

In CHM, where the karyotype is 46XX the chromosomes are entirely of paternal origin due to fertilisation of an anuclear egg by a haploid (23X) sperm which then duplicates its own chromosomes. The mitochondrial DNA is of maternal origin. When the karyotype in CHM is 46XY, all chromosomes are of paternal origin resulting from dispermy. In contrast, the extra haploid complement of chromosomes in the triploid composition in PHM is derived from the father. The fetus in a partial mole generally has stigmata of triploidy, including growth restriction and multiple congenital anomalies.

Table 5.1 Features of partial and complete hydatidiform moles (adapted from *Obstetrics & Gynecology* 104 (6), American College of Obstetricians and Gynecologists, ACOG Practice Bulletin No. 53: Diagnosis and Treatment of gestational trophoblastic disease, 1365–77, 2004)[1]

Features	Complete mole	Partial mole
Pathology		
Karyotype	Most commonly 46XX (90%) or 46XY (10%)	Most commonly 69XXX, or 69 XXY
Fetal or embryonic tissue	Absent	Present
Amnion, fetal red blood cells	Absent	Usually present
Hydropic change of villi	Focal	Diffuse
Trophoblastic proliferation	Focal	Diffuse
Trophoblastic stromal inclusions	Absent	Present
Implantation-site trophoblast	Absent	Present
Clinical presentation		
Diagnosis	Molar gestation	Missed miscarriage
Uterine size	Can be larger for gestational age	Small for gestational age
Theca lutein cysts	15–25%	Rare
Medical complications	Less than 25%	Rare
Postmolar malignant sequelae	6–32%	< 5%
Hyperemesis	Common	Less common
Hyperthyroidism	Rare but can happen	Very rare
Early onset pre-eclampsia	Rare but can happen	Very rare

Presentation and diagnosis

COMPLETE AND PARTIAL HYDATIDIFORM MOLE

Since the advent of high-resolution ultrasound and the ability to quantify serum hCG, the presentation of these disorders has changed dramatically. Vaginal bleeding remains the most common presenting symptom and is seen in about 90% of cases. Now that most CHM are identified in the first trimester, the other signs and symptoms such as excessive uterine enlargement, theca lutein cysts, hyperemesis, pre-eclampsia, hyperthyroidism and respiratory difficulties are less commonly seen. PHM typically presents as a missed or incomplete miscarriage and the diagnosis is usually only made after histological examination of the specimen.

The marked swelling of chorionic villi in CHM produces a characteristic vesicular sonographic pattern often referred to as 'snow storm' appearance. However, it is more difficult to distinguish an early complete mole from degenerating chorionic tissue, since small molar chorionic villi in the first trimester may be difficult to visualise on ultrasound. The average diameter of the largest, most hydropic villi, is significantly greater in cases of CHM and PHM detected by ultrasound examination in the first trimester compared to the diameter of those not detected sonographically but beyond 14 weeks such differences are minimal. These findings suggest that, although sonographer expertise could potentially increase ultrasound detection rates somewhat for PHM and CHM, a significant proportion of cases demonstrate minimal hydropic change in the first trimester and are therefore likely to remain unidentifiable by ultrasound examination prior to evacuation, even with improved sonographer expertise. Thus, histological assessment of material obtained from the medical or surgical management of all failed pregnancies is recommended, to exclude trophoblastic neoplasia.[2]

However, histological distinction between CHM and non-molar products of miscarriage in early pregnancy can be very difficult because many features of normal and molar placentas may appear to be similar in the early weeks, particularly around 6 weeks of gestation. In difficult cases, immunostaining, together with cytogenetic analysis, can help to distinguish early CHM from other first-trimester losses that can have hydropic villous changes; for example, hydropic miscarriages and trisomy.[4]

The distinction between hydatidiform mole and missed miscarriage before surgical evacuation can be improved by correlating the ultrasonographic findings with serum hCG levels. hCG levels greater than two multiples of median may help.[2] Some authors reported that pre-evacuation hCG values were commonly found to be greater than 100 000 miu/ml.[3] Women with PHM less commonly present with such high levels of hCG as in CHM.

In PHM, two sonographic findings are commonly associated with the diagnosis: focal cystic changes in the placenta and a ratio of the transverse to anteroposterior dimension of the gestational sac greater than 1.5. Changes in the shape of the gestational sac may be part of the embryopathy of triploidy. When both findings are detectable, the positive predictive value for PHM approaches 90%. Ultrasound may also show the presence of a growth-restricted fetus with multiple congenital anomalies associated with a focally hydropic placenta.[3]

GESTATIONAL TROPHOBLASTIC NEOPLASIA

The clinical presentation of malignant GTD is more important in determining treatment and outcome that the precise histological diagnosis. Non-metastatic GTN or locally invasive mole develops in 15% of women following evacuation of CHM and infrequently after other gestations.[3] It is characterised by invasion of the myometrium, which can lead to perforation of the myometrium, producing intraperitoneal bleeding or erode into uterine vessels, causing vaginal haemorrhage. A bulky necrotic tumour may also serve as a nidus for infection.

Gestational choriocarcinomas are derived from term pregnancies in 50% of cases, with equal portions of the remaining 50% from histologically normal gestations and hydatidiform moles. It is a malignancy comprising both neoplastic syncytiotrophoblast and cytotrophoblast elements without chorionic villi. Gestational choriocarcinomas tend to develop early systemic metastasis, most commonly to the vagina, lung, liver and brain, and chemotherapy is indicated when it is diagnosed histologically. In some of these cases, gynaecological symptoms may be minimal or absent and the antecedent pregnancy may be remote in time. The presenting symptoms may be varied, owing to distant metastasis; for example, dyspnoea, chest pain, haemoptysis, vomiting, seizures, headache and visual disturbance. Such cases can be diagnostically challenging but a combination of gynaecological history and elevated serum hCG usually makes the diagnosis clear. Biopsy should be avoided because of risk of haemorrhage. Vaginal metastasis may present with irregular bleeding or purulent discharge and are most commonly located in the fornices or suburethrally. Vaginal metastases are highly vascular and biopsy of vaginal metastases should be absolutely avoided. The desire to avoid haemorrhage should supersede the interest of obtaining an unequivocal pathological diagnosis.

PSTT are the least common type of GTD comprising less than 2% of all cases. PSTT most commonly occurs following a normal pregnancy but can also occur after a non-molar miscarriage or a complete hydatidiform mole and very rarely following a partial mole. The average interval between the prior pregnancy and presentation of PSTT is 3.4 years, which is much longer than the interval for occurrence of the more common types of trophoblastic diseases. The most frequent presentation is bleeding following amenorrhea and the hCG level, while elevated, is characteristically lower for the volume of disease than in the other types of GTD. The tumour is diploid and arises from the nonvillous trophoblast and the pathology is characterised by intermediate trophoblastic cells with vacuolated cytoplasm, the expression of placental alkaline phosphatase rather than hCG and the absence of cytotrophoblast and villi. Although in most women the disease is confined to the uterus, clinical presentation of PSTT can range from slow-growing disease limited to the uterus to more rapidly growing metastatic disease that is similar in behaviour to choriocarcinoma.

Management of molar pregnancy

Suction curettage is the preferred method of evacuation regardless of uterine size. During dilatation of the cervix, there might be brisk uterine bleeding owing to the passage of retained blood. Soon after commencing the procedure, uterine bleeding is generally well controlled and the uterus rapidly regresses in size. In case of PHM, suction curettage may become difficult or impossible because of the size of fetal parts. Under such circumstances medical evacuation can be used. Medical evacuation of CHM should be avoided if possible, because of concerns about the use of potent oxytocic agents and the risk of dissemination of trophoblastic tissue emboli through the venous system. However, there is little supporting evidence to substantiate such concerns. Evacuation of the uterine cavity is usually performed under general anaesthesia but local or regional anaesthesia may be used for a woman who has a small uterus. Intravenous oxytocin infusion before completion of evacuation of molar tissue is not recommended. Where

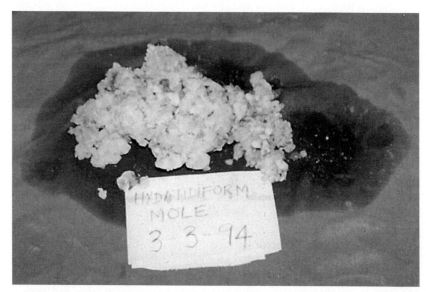

Figure 5.1 Macroscopic appearance of hydatidiform mole evacuated at 18 weeks gestation, resembling a bunch of grapes

significant haemorrhage takes place before completion of evacuation, oxytocin infusion may be used and can be continued for several hours postoperatively. Although preparation of the cervix immediately prior to evacuation of a mole is safe, prolonged cervical preparation, particularly with prostaglandins, should be avoided where possible, to reduce the risk of embolisation of trophoblastic tissue.

There are conflicting views about administration of anti-D immunoglobulin after the evacuation of molar tissue. The American College of Obstetrics and Gynecology recommends its administration, even though fetal blood cells should not be present in a complete mole.[1] The RCOG guideline states that anti-D prophylaxis is not required in CHM.[2] In case of PHM, anti-D prophylaxis should be given after evacuation because of the presence of fetal red blood cells in the conceptus.

Pulmonary complications may occur around the time of evacuation of a molar pregnancy among women with a markedly enlarged uterus. Trophoblastic embolisation is quoted as one of the common causes for respiratory distress. Other possible causes are high-output congestive heart failure due to anaemia, hyperthyroidism, pre-eclampsia or iatrogenic fluid overload. Hyperthyroidism and pregnancy-induced hypertension usually abate promptly after evacuation of the mole and may not require specific therapy. Theca lutein cysts may take several months to resolve after evacuation of molar tissue but very rarely need to be removed. Surgical intervention should be reserved for rupture or torsion of ovary, which is rare.

In carefully selected women who do not wish to preserve childbearing capacity, hysterectomy may be an alternative form of treatment. It reduces the risk of GTN when compared with suction curettage. However, the risk of post-molar GTN after hysterectomy remains approximately 3–5% and these women should be monitored postoperatively with serial hCG estimation.

Follow-up after GTD

After evacuation of a molar pregnancy it is important to monitor all women carefully to diagnose and treat malignant sequelae promptly. All women diagnosed with GTD should be provided with written information about the condition and the need for referral for follow-up to a trophoblastic screening centre should be explained. Registration of women with GTD represents a minimum standard of care. After registration, follow-up consists of serial estimation of hCG levels, either in blood or urine specimens. Quantitative serum hCG determination should be performed using commercially available assays capable of detecting beta-hCG to baseline values of less than 5 miu/ml. If hCG falls to normal within 8 weeks of evacuation, monitoring can be stopped at 6 months post-evacuation. If the hCG falls more slowly, monitoring can stop at 6 months after the first normal value after normalisation. After normalisation of the serum hCG, monitoring is by urine hCG. This means that pregnancy should be avoided for a minimum of 6 months after hCG levels returns to normal.

All women are advised to avoid the use of estrogen-containing oral contraceptive pills while hCG levels are elevated, as there is a theoretical risk of inducing metastatic or drug-resistant disease. Intrauterine contraceptive devices should not be inserted until the hCG normalises, because of the risk of uterine perforation, bleeding and infection if residual tumour is present. Barrier methods of contraception are advisable until hCG levels revert to normal. There is no evidence as to whether single agent progestogens have any effect on GTN. The combined oral contraceptive pill may be used after the hCG levels have returned to normal. If oral contraception has been started before the diagnosis of GTD is made, the woman can be advised to continue but she should be advised that there is a potential but small increased risk of developing GTN.

Women with prior partial or complete moles have a ten-fold increased risk (1–2% incidence) of a second hydatidiform mole in a subsequent pregnancy. Therefore, all future pregnancies should be evaluated by early obstetric ultrasonography. All women should notify the screening centre at the end of any future pregnancy, whatever the outcome of the pregnancy. hCG levels are measured 6–8 weeks after the end of the pregnancy to exclude disease recurrence.

Management of GTN

There is no role for chemotherapy if serum hCG levels keep decreasing after evacuation of a molar pregnancy. The diagnosis of malignant sequelae, as indicated by the need for chemotherapy, include the plateau or increase of hCG levels after evacuation of hydatidiform mole, the histological diagnosis of choriocarcinoma or invasive mole on the basis of findings from uterine curettage or identification of clinical or radiographic evidence of metastases. Repeat curettage is not recommended because it does not often induce remission or influence treatment and it may result in uterine perforation and haemorrhage.

To diagnose post-molar trophoblastic disease, the International Federation of Gynecology and Obstetrics (FIGO) has recommended standardised hCG criteria. Based on Consensus Committee recommendations from the Society of Gynecologic Oncology, the International Society for the Study of Trophoblastic Disease and the International

Gynecologic Cancer Society, the following criteria were proposed by FIGO:[5]

1. an hCG level plateau of four values plus or minus 10% recorded over a 3-week period (days 1,7,14 and 21)
2. an hCG level increase of more than 10% of three values recorded over a 2-week period (days 1,7 and 14)
3. persistence of detectable hCG for more than 6 months after molar evacuation.

If hCG values do not fall as expected, a new intrauterine pregnancy should be excluded on the basis of hCG levels and ultrasonography, especially when there has been a long delay in follow-up of serial hCG levels and noncompliance with contraception.

To allow objective comparison of reported information as well as of treatment results, FIGO reports data on GTN using an anatomical staging system (Table 5.2).[3] Stage 4 tumours generally have the histological pattern of choriocarcinoma and commonly follow a non-molar pregnancy, with protracted delays in diagnosis and large tumour burdens.

To predict the likelihood of drug resistance and to assist in selecting appropriate chemotherapy, a modified WHO prognostic scoring system was recommended by FIGO in 2000 (Table 5.3).[6] In general, women with stage-1 disease have a low-risk score and women with stage-4 disease have a high risk score. Thus, the distinction between low and high risk applies to stages 2 and 3.

Women are assessed before chemotherapy using the modified WHO scoring system. Women with scores less than or equal to 6 are at low risk and are treated with single-agent intramuscular methotrexate alternating daily with folinic acid for 1 week followed by 6 rest days. Women with scores more than or equal to 7 are at high risk and are

Table 5.2	FIGO anatomical staging for gestational trophoblastic neoplasia (GTN)	
GTN stage	Description
1	Disease confined to uterus; persistently elevated hCG
2	GTN extends outside of the uterus but is limited to the genital structures (adnexa, vagina, broad ligament)
3	GTN extends to the lungs, with or without known genital tract involvement
4	Far advanced disease with involvement of the brain, liver, kidneys or gastrointestinal tract

Table 5.3 Modified World Health Organization prognostic scoring system as adapted by FIGO (2000)[5]

Scores	0	1	2	4
Age	< 40 years	> 40 years	–	–
Antecedent pregnancy	mole	abortion	term	–
Interval months from index pregnancy	< 4	4 – < 7	7 – < 13	± 13
Pretreatment serum hCG (iu/l)	< 1000	> 10 000	< 100 000	> 100 000
Largest tumour size, including uterus (cm)	< 3	3 – < 5	± 5	–
Site of metastases	lung	spleen/kidney	gastrointestinal	liver/brain
Metastases (n)	–	1–4	5–8	> 8
Previous failed chemotherapy	–	–	single drug	2 or more drugs

treated with intravenous multi-agent chemotherapy, which includes combinations of methotrexate, dactinomycin, etoposide, cyclophosphamide and vincristine. Treatment is continued in all cases until the hCG level has returned to normal and then for a further 6 consecutive weeks. The need for chemotherapy following a CHM is 15% and 0.5% after a PHM. The development of postpartum GTN requiring chemotherapy occurs at a rate of 1/50 000 births. The cure rate for women with a score of less than or equal to 6 is almost 100% and for those with a score of 7 or more is 95%.[2]

PSTTs are rare and are generally not sensitive to chemotherapy as other forms of malignant GTD. It is thus important to distinguish these tumours histologically. They are characterised by the absence of villi with proliferation of intermediate trophoblast cells. The number of syncytiotrophoblast cells observed is decreased in PSTT, with relatively lower levels of hCG secreted by these tumours. Surgery is an important modality in the treatment of PSTT and, fortunately, most women have disease confined to the uterus and are cured by hysterectomy.

Women who undergo chemotherapy should be advised not to conceive for 1 year after completion of treatment. In women who conceive within 12 months of completing chemotherapy, there may be an increased risk of miscarriage, a higher rate of termination of pregnancy and an increased rate of stillbirth compared with the normal population.[2]

Following completion of chemotherapy for GTN, once hCG remission has been achieved, women should undergo serial determinations of hCG levels at 2-week intervals for the first 3 months of remission and then at 1-month intervals until monitoring has shown 1 year of normal hCG levels. The risk of recurrence after 1 year of remission is less than 1% but late recurrences have been observed rarely. Women should be advised to use a reliable form of hormonal contraception during the first year of remission.[1]

Management of hydatidiform mole and a co-existent fetus

Both complete and partial moles with co-existent fetuses have been reported. This condition occurs in 1/22 000–1/100 000 pregnancies. Most of these pregnancies are diagnosed antepartum by ultrasound findings of a complex, cystic placental component distinct from the fetoplacental unit but, in some cases, the diagnosis is not suspected until examination of the placenta following delivery. Complications of hydatidiform mole with a co-existent fetus appear to be increased and include hyperthyroidism, haemorrhage, preterm labour and pregnancy-induced hypertension. In some studies, compared with singleton hydatidiform moles, twin pregnancies with a fetus and a mole were found to carry an increased risk for post-molar GTD with a higher proportion of women having metastatic disease and requiring multi-agent chemotherapy.[1]

There are no clear guidelines for the management of this condition, so advice should be sought from the regional fetal medicine unit and the relevant trophoblastic screening centre. The ultrasound examination should be repeated to exclude retroplacental haematoma, other placental abnormalities or degenerating myoma, and to fully evaluate the fetoplacental unit for evidence of a partial mole or gross fetal malformations. If the diagnosis is still suspected and continuation of pregnancy is desired, fetal karyotyping should be considered. A chest X-ray may be also considered to screen for metastases and serial serum hCG values monitored. After delivery, the placenta should be histologically evaluated and the mother followed closely with serial hCG values, similar to the management of a singleton hydatidiform mole.

Key points

• Trophoblastic disease can occur as a locally invasive entity or as metastatic disease.

- Partial and complete hydatidiform moles are distinct disease processes.
- GTN can occur following partial or complete hydatidiform mole and hence meticulous follow-up of benign disease is essential.
- Treatment of GTN results in high cure rates.

References

1. American College of Obstetricians and Gynecologists. ACOG Practice Bulletin No. 53: Diagnosis and treatment of gestational trophoblastic disease. *Obstet Gynecol* 2004;103:1365–77.
2. Royal College of Obstetricians and Gynaecologists. *The Management of Gestational Trophoblastic Disease*. Green-top Guideline No. 38. London: RCOG; 2010 [www.rcog.org.uk/womens-health/clinical-guidance/management-gestational-trophoblastic-neoplasia-green-top-38].
3. Berkowitz RS, Goldstein DP. Current management of gestational trophoblastic diseases. *Gynecol Oncol* 2009;112:654–62.
4. Lash GE, Quenby S, Burton GJ, Nakashima A, Kamat BR, Ray J, et al. Gestational diseases – a workshop report. *Placenta* 2008;29 Suppl A:S92–4.
5. Kohorn EI. The new FIGO 2000 staging and risk factor scoring system for gestational trophoblastic disease: description and clinical assessment. *Int J Gynecol Cancer* 2001;11:73–7.
6. International Federation of Gynecology and Obstetrics Oncology Committee. FIGO staging for gestational trophoblastic neoplasia 2000. *Int J Gynecol Obstet* 2002;77: 285–7.

6 Hyperemesis gravidarum

Nausea and vomiting are very common in pregnancy and affect up to 85% of pregnant women.[1] Although commonly known as 'morning sickness' very few women experience nausea solely in the morning and majority (80%) report nausea throughout the day. The condition is usually mild and self-limiting and usually resolves by 14 weeks of gestation. Hyperemesis gravidarum, however, is unexplained intractable form of nausea and vomiting in pregnancy leading to fluid, electrolyte imbalance and weight loss. This condition affects 0.3–2.0% of pregnant women and is one of the most common reasons for hospitalisation in the first trimester of pregnancy.[2] The Confidential Enquiries into Maternal Deaths in the United Kingdom 1991–1993 reported three maternal deaths related to hyperemesis.[3] Fortunately, there has been no recorded mortality attributable to hyperemesis gravidarum in the two most recent reports.

Diagnosis

Hyperemesis gravidarum is often diagnosed subjectively based on the symptoms of severe nausea and vomiting leading to dehydration, fluid and electrolyte imbalance, nutritional deficiency and often necessitating hospitalisation. While a criterion of weight loss of more than 5% of prepregnancy weight has been used as a standard for diagnosis, the Fairweather criteria define hyperemesis gravidarum as more than three episodes of vomiting in a day with weight loss, ketonaemia, electrolyte imbalance and volume depletion, with onset usually at 4–8 weeks of pregnancy.[4,5] According to the International Classification of Diseases (ICD-10), hyperemesis gravidarum is defined as persistent and excessive vomiting with onset before 22 completed weeks of gestation and is subclassified as mild and severe (Table 6.1).[5]

Table 6.1 ICD-10 subclassification of hyperemesis gravidarum	
Sub-class	Description
021.0 Mild hyperemesis gravidarum	Hyperemesis gravidarum, mild or unspecified, starting before the end of 22nd week of gestation
021.1 Hyperemesis gravidarum with metabolic disturbance	Hyperemesis gravidarum starting before the end of 22nd week of gestation, with metabolic disturbance; e.g. carbohydrate depletion, dehydration and electrolyte imbalance

Aetiology

Although the precise cause for hyperemesis gravidarum remains unknown, various aetiological factors have been proposed. Human chorionic gonadotrophin (hCG) is the most commonly cited endocrine factor based on the observation that the symptoms tend to mirror the rise and fall of serum hCG and are therefore related to the placental mass. This is supported by the fact that hyperemesis gravidarum is more commonly observed in molar pregnancies and multiple pregnancies which have a higher placental mass and higher hCG levels. In a review of the 15 published studies (1990–2004), 11 showed significantly higher concentration of serum hCG in women with hyperemesis compared with controls.[6] It is proposed that hCG, being structurally similar to thyroid-stimulating hormone (TSH) stimulates thyroid function and contributes to hyperemesis. Hyperemesis gravidarum is more commonly associated with the presence of a female fetus and high levels of maternal estradiol concentration are also hypothesised to be a contributory factor for severe nausea and vomiting in pregnancy.[7] Although various psychosocial issues have been linked with hyperemesis, more recent studies have suggested the psychosocial symptoms to be the result of stress arising from hyperemesis gravidarum rather than being causative.[8]

Predisposing factors

Symptoms of nausea and vomiting in pregnancy are more common in:

• younger women
• women who experience nausea and vomiting while taking the combined contraceptive pill
• women with a history of motion sickness

- women with a history of migraines
- women carrying a female fetus
- women with a genetic predisposition: explained by the fact that sisters and mothers of women affected with hyperemesis gravidarum are more likely to be affected themselves with the condition.[9] Higher concordance among monozygotic twins also provides evidence for a genetic component to hyperemesis gravidarum.[2]

In contrast, smoking and higher body mass index have been associated with a reduction in the risk of hyperemesis gravidarum.[10]

Diagnosis and investigation

Hyperemesis gravidarum is a diagnosis of exclusion and other potential causes of nausea and vomiting should be excluded. Investigations should include:

- urine dipstick test (especially for ketonuria) and midstream urine test to exclude urinary tract infection
- urea and electrolytes (hyponatraemia, hypokalaemia, low serum urea may be observed)
- full blood count and haematocrit (raised haematocrit may be observed signifying dehydration)
- liver function tests (mildly elevated liver enzymes may be seen in almost 50% of women with hyperemesis gravidarum and this is thought to be contributed by temporary impairment of mitochondrial fatty acid oxidation)
- thyroid function tests (low TSH and high thyroxine levels may be observed in approximately two-thirds of women with hyperemesis gravidarum as a result of biochemical hyperthyroidism, owing to the thyroid-stimulant effect of hCG. This is usually self-limiting and does not require any further investigation or treatment unless it fails to resolve with improvement in symptoms of hyperemesis gravidarum. Gestational thyrotoxicosis is more commonly seen in women from an Asian background)[11]
- ultrasound scan to exclude molar pregnancy or multiple pregnancy.

Differential diagnosis

The list of differential diagnoses can be long and includes a whole range of conditions such as hyperthyroidism, hyperparathyroidism, diabetic ketoacidosis, gastroenteritis, biliary tract disease, peptic ulceration, hepatitis, appendicitis, pancreatitis, pyelonephritis, ovarian cyst accident, renal stones, migraine, drug toxicity, acute fatty liver of pregnancy and very-early-onset pre-eclampsia. Onset of symptoms antedating pregnancy or after 9 weeks of gestation or association with symptoms of abdominal pain and pyrexia are suggestive of causes other than hyperemesis gravidarum.

Complications

MATERNAL COMPLICATIONS

Maternal complications of hyperemesis gravidarum include:

- Wernicke's encephalopathy owing to thiamine (vitamin B1) deficiency: a rare but serious condition which commonly presents as confusion or simple apathy but may present as ataxia, nystagmus and dementia (classic diagnostic triad). Occasionally, infusion of dextrose solutions may precipitate encephalopathy in the presence of thiamine deficiency
- electrolyte imbalance: hyponatraemia (plasma sodium less than 120 mmol/l) may present as lethargy, seizures and respiratory arrest. Central pontine myelinolysis (spastic quadraparesis, pseudobulbar palsy and impaired consciousness) may be precipitated by severe hyponatraemia or even its rapid correction[12]
- liver failure
- renal failure
- Mallory–Weiss tears of the oesophagus
- oesophageal rupture
- retinal detachment
- pneumomediastinum
- maternal death: uncommon but rarely may occur following hyperemesis gravidarum or as a result of intervention.

FETAL COMPLICATIONS

Adverse infant outcomes such as low Apgar scores, low birth weight, small for gestational age and preterm births are mostly limited to women with poor maternal weight gain owing to hyperemesis.[13]

Management

Hyperemesis gravidarum is a debilitating condition and women not only need a careful and individual assessment and care plan for the management of their symptoms but also require significant support from practitioners and their family. Mild forms of nausea and vomiting are usually managed by general lifestyle and dietary advice in the form of smaller frequent meals with sufficient small amounts of fluids and avoiding a fat rich diet. Light snacks in the form of nuts, dry salty biscuits and cold food may be helpful for some. Providing emotional support and offering supportive counselling may be helpful on occasions as women often feel unsupported and seek help from healthcare professionals who may have a tendency to overlook their symptoms as normal part of pregnancy.

If, however, symptoms cannot be managed with general lifestyle and dietary measures alone, medication may be recommended. There is no licensed medication for the treatment of nausea and vomiting in pregnancy in the UK and, as yet, no approved evidence-based guidance on its management. The National Institute for Health and Clinical Excellence (NICE) guidance on antenatal care, however, recommends that, if a woman requests or would like to consider treatment for nausea and vomiting in pregnancy, there are interventions which appear to be effective in reducing the severity of symptoms.[14]

NON-PHARMACOLOGICAL INTERVENTIONS

Ginger

Ginger 1 g/day has no known teratogenic effects and is available as tea, biscuits, crystals or sugared ginger cubes.

P6 acupressure either manually or with elasticated bands

The P6 Neiguan point is on the inside of the wrist, about two to three finger-breadths proximal to the wrist crease between the tendons, about 1 cm deep. Manual pressure is applied to this point for 5 minutes every 4 hours or by wearing an elasticated band with a 1-cm round plastic protruding button centred over the P6 point.[15]

Pyridoxine

Pyridoxine (vitamin B6) administered orally at a dose of 10–25 mg three times a day has been proven to be more effective than placebo for severe nausea and is well tolerated.

Self-help

NICE recommends that information about all forms of self-help and non-pharmacological treatments should be made available for pregnant woman with nausea and vomiting.[14]

PHARMACOLOGICAL TREATMENT

Antihistamines may be used. Hospitalisation and correction of dehydration with intravenous fluids may be required in women with severe symptoms with or without significant ketonuria. Certain predisposing factors amongst women with HG requiring hospital admissions have been identified (Table 6.2). Physiological (0.9%) saline or Hartmann solution is the fluid of choice for replacement. Double-strength saline solutions should, however, be avoided owing to the potential risk of precipitating central pontine myelinolysis by rapid correction of hyponatraemia.[12] Potassium chloride may be administered as an additive with each bag of saline or as a ready-mixed solution of 0.9% saline with 40 mmol/l of potassium. Dextrose infusions should be avoided as these can precipitate Wernicke's encephalopathy. Total food abstinence may be necessary to break the symptom cycle in addition to antiemetics.

Antiemetics are superior to placebo in reducing symptoms and judicious usage of antiemetic medications may prove beneficial in reducing significant morbidity associated with hyperemesis gravidarum. Commonly prescribed antiemetics include cyclizine (oral, intramuscular or intravenous) 50 mg three times a day or promethazine (oral) 25 mg once at bedtime or prochlorperazine orally 5 mg three times a day or 12.5 mg twice or thrice daily intramuscularly or metoclopramide (oral, intramuscular or subcutaneous) in a dose of 10 mg three to four

Table 6.2 **Risk factors for hospital admission for hyperemesis gravidarum[5] (reprinted from *Best Practice & Research: Clinical Gastroenterology* 21 (5), Ismail SK and Kenny L, Review on hyperemesis gravidarum, 755–69 (2007), with permission from Elsevier)**

Risk factor	Relative risk
Previous hyperemesis	29
Hyperthyroidism	4.5
Psychiatric illness	4.1
Previous molar pregnancy	3.3
Multiple gestations:	
multiple male and female	3.7
multiple males	2.4
multiple females	1.7
Pre-existing diabetes mellitus	2.6
Gastrointestinal disorders	2.5
Asthma	1.5
Maternal age less than 20 years	1.5

times a day or chlorpromazine 10–25 mg three times a day orally or 25 mg three times a day intramuscularly.

For persistent symptoms, the 5-HT3 receptor antagonist, ondansetron (4–8 mg) may be effective. Steroids in the form of intravenous hydrocortisone (100 mg twice daily) followed by oral prednisolone 40 mg daily may be used in refractory cases; these are considered to be safe in pregnancy. In addition, antacids in the form of ranitidine or omeprazole may be used for symptoms of dyspepsia.

Thiamine (vitamin B1) supplementation should be considered in cases of persistent hyperemesis gravidarum to prevent Wernicke's encephalopathy. This could be in the form of oral thiamine hydrochloride tablet 25–50 mg three times a day or intravenous thiamine 100 mg in 100 ml 0.9% saline as a slow once-weekly infusion.

Diazepam, on its own or in combination with antiemetic therapy, has been shown to reduce the need for hospitalisation but dependency and potential adverse fetal effects are a cause for concern.

Thromboprophylaxis should be offered to women hospitalised for hyperemesis gravidarum. Total parenteral nutrition may be considered necessary in highly refractory cases but this should only be used as a last resort owing to the potential complications such as thrombosis, infection and metabolic disturbances.

In exceptional circumstances when all modalities of treatment fail to control the symptoms and maternal life is under treat, termination of pregnancy may be seen as the only definitive cure.

Conclusion

Hyperemesis gravidarum is a poorly understood condition and early recognition of the condition is vital for optimal management. Treatment should be multimodal, with general lifestyle measures to ensure adequate hydration and prevention of complications. Hyperemesis gravidarum is not only associated with maternal morbidity but is also known to increase the risk of prematurity and small-for-gestational age fetuses. Preterm birth rates up to three times higher have been observed in women with weight gain of less than 7 kg compared with those with weight gain of 7 kg or more.[13]

A risk of recurrence of approximately 15.2% has been quoted for women who have experienced hyperemesis gravidarum in their first pregnancy.[5] There is some evidence to suggest that pre-emptive medical treatment with oral antiemetics in women with a history of severe hyperemesis gravidarum may be of some benefit in reducing the severity of symptoms in the current pregnancy; in turn, this could reduce the risk of hospital admission and the consequences thereof.[16,17]

Key points

- Hyperemesis gravidarum affects 0.3–2.0% of pregnant women and is one of the most common causes of hospitalisation in the first trimester of pregnancy.
- Early recognition of hyperemesis gravidarum is recommended to prevent serious morbidity.
- In addition to general lifestyle measures, antiemetics and intravenous fluids remain the mainstay of management.

References

1. Gadsby R, Barnie-Adshead AM, Jagger C. A prospective study of nausea and vomiting during pregnancy. *Br J Gen Practice* 1992;43:245–8.
2. Goodwin TM. Hyperemesis gravidarum. *Obstet Gynecol Clin N Am* 2008;35:401–17.
3. Department of Health. *Report on Confidential Enquiries into Maternal Deaths in the United Kingdom 1991–1993*. London: TSO; 1996.
4. Jueckstock JK, Kaestner R, Mylonas I. Managing hyperemesis gravidarum: a multimodal challenge. *BMC Med* 2010;8:46 [doi:10.1186/1741-7015-8-46].
5. Ismail SK, Kenny L. Review on hyperemesis gravidarum. *Best Pract Res Clin Gastroenterol* 2007;21(5):755–69.
6. Verberg MF, Gilliott DJ, Al-Fardan N, Grudzinkas JG. Hyperemesis gravidarum, a literature review. *Hum Reprod Update* 2005;11:527–39.
7. Lagiou P, Tamimi R, Mucci LA, Trichopoulos D, Adami HO, Hsieh CC. Nausea and vomiting in pregnancy in relation to prolactin, estrogens and progesterone: a prospective study. *Obstet Gynecol* 2003;101:639–44.
8. Swallow BL, Lindow SW, Masson EA, Hay DM. Psychosocial health in early pregnancy; relationship with nausea and vomiting. *J Obstet Gynecol* 2004;24:28–32.
9. Zhang Y, Cantor RM, Macgibbon K, Romero R, Goodwin TM, et al. Familial aggregation of hyperemesis gravidarum. *Am J Obstet Gynecol* 2011;204:230.e1–7.
10. Bailit JL. Hyperemesis gravidarum: epidemiologic findings from a large cohort. *Am J Obstet Gynecol* 2005;193:811–14.
11. Price A, Davies R, Heller SR, Milford-Ward A, Weetman AP. Asian women are at increased risk of gestational thyrotoxicosis. *J Clin Endocrinol Metab* 1996;81:1160–3.
12. Neill AM, Nelson-Piercy C. Hyperemesis gravidarum. *The Obstetrician and Gynaecologist* 2003;5:204–7.
13. Dodds L, Fell DB, Joseph KS, Allen VM, Butler B. Outcomes of pregnancies complicated by hyperemesis gravidarum. *Obstet Gynecol* 2006;107:285–92.
14. National Institute for Health and Clinical Excellence. *Antenatal Care: Routine Care for the Healthy Pregnant Woman*. Clinical Guideline 62. London: NICE; 2008 [www.nice.org.uk/CG062].
15. Sheehan P. Hyperemesis gravidarum: assessment and management. *Aust Fam Physician* 2007;36:698–701.
16. Koren G, Maltepe C. Pre-emptive therapy for severe nausea and vomiting of pregnancy and hyperemesis gravidarum. *J Obstet Gynaecol* 2004;24:530–3.
17. Gadsby R, Barnie-Adshead T. Severe nausea and vomiting of pregnancy: should it be treated with appropriate pharmacotherapy? *The Obstetrician & Gynaecologist*, 2011;13:107–11.

7 Abdominal and pelvic pain in early pregnancy

Abdominal pain in early pregnancy brings fear and uncertainty to every expectant mother and hence most women will present sooner to health professionals than if they were not pregnant. Early pregnancy is defined here as the period from conception to the end of first trimester. As such the primary concern in the mind of a gravid woman in such circumstances is that of miscarriage or an ectopic pregnancy. It is important to remember, however, that abdominopelvic pain, although common during early pregnancy, may accompany serious or minor disorders and includes conditions which are not directly related to pregnancy.

Many pregnant women presenting with pain are seen in an early pregnancy assessment unit and will result in a diagnosis of threatened, inevitable, incomplete or complete miscarriage or, in some cases, an ectopic pregnancy. Some of these cases present with complaints of vaginal bleeding, which most often serves as an indicator of the possible cause.

Apart from other medical or surgical causes, sepsis can also lead to abdominopelvic pain. The eighth report of the Confidential Enquiries into Maternal Deaths in the UK (2006–2008) reported 29 deaths from genital tract sepsis, of which seven were in early pregnancy (arising before 24 completed weeks of gestation). Two women died from septic miscarriage and two after a termination of pregnancy. In this report, there were eighty-eight indirect maternal deaths from causes other than cardiac disease. Nine of these were due to disease of the gastrointestinal tract, of which two were from complications of duodenal ulcer.

General principles of management

Women with abdominopelvic pain in early pregnancy may present at the early pregnancy assessment unit or the accident and emergency department. Irrespective of their history of amenorrhoea, contraception or bleeding, all women in the reproductive age group complaining of abdominal or pelvic pain should have a sensitive urinary pregnancy test done at the time of their presentation to exclude pregnancy-related causes. Problems directly related to pregnancy, such as miscarriage (see Chapter 2) and ectopic pregnancy (see Chapter 4), have been dealt with in the relevant chapters of this book and will not be discussed here.

Abdominopelvic pain is a manifestation of acute abdomen and should be dealt with promptly and, if necessary, emergency surgical intervention must be considered to avoid miscarriage, maternal morbidity and mortality. The approach to pregnant women with severe abdominal pain is very similar to that for nonpregnant women with acute abdomen. However, the physiological changes associated with pregnancy must be considered when interpreting findings from the history and physical examination.

Clearly, the case of a pregnant woman with acute abdomen is a clinical scenario that overlaps different specialties. So, in such cases it is important to consider involving a general surgical specialist, a specialist in maternal-fetal medicine as well as an obstetrician and gynaecologist. A cause for acute abdomen can occur coincidentally with pregnancy. Some clinical conditions are more likely to occur in pregnancy and some others are specific to pregnancy. Hence, a wide range of possible differential diagnoses should be considered.

Differential diagnoses

Causes of pelvic pain during early pregnancy may be obstetric, non-obstetric genitourinary or non-gynaecological.

OBSTETRIC

The most common obstetric cause is spontaneous miscarriage (threatened, inevitable, incomplete, complete, septic or missed) and the most common serious obstetric cause is ectopic gestation (ruptured or unruptured). These disorders have been dealt with in other chapters of this book.

NON-OBSTETRIC GENITOURINARY

Non-obstetric genitourinary causes include:

- ovarian cyst rupture
- adnexal torsion
- ureteric obstruction (including calculus)
- acute pyelonephritis

- acute cystitis
- ovarian hyperstimulation syndrome (OHSS).

NON-GYNAECOLOGICAL CAUSES

Non-gynaecological causes include:

- acute pancreatitis
- acute appendicitis
- acute cholecystitis
- peptic ulcer
- bowel obstruction or perforation
- peptic ulcer
- gastroenteritis
- meckel's diverticulitis
- pancreatic pseudocyst
- mesenteric venous thrombosis
- splenic artery aneurysm
- acute intermittent porphyria
- sickle cell disease.

Clinical approach to diagnosis

HISTORY

A detailed history should be elicited about the time and type of onset of pain, its duration, intensity, character and any associated symptoms. The characteristics of pain vary with different aetiologies. It is also important to ascertain the following facts about the pain:

Is there any relation to eating a meal?
Did the pain awaken the woman from sleep?
Is it localised and has the location changed?
Is it associated with nausea and vomiting?
Does anything make the pain better or worse?

PHYSIOLOGICAL BASIS OF CLINICAL FEATURES

Findings from clinical examination may be less prominent compared with those of nonpregnant women with the same disorder. Peritoneal signs are often absent in pregnancy because of the lifting and stretching of the anterior abdominal wall. This phenomenon often means that the underlying inflammation has no direct contact with the parietal peritoneum which precludes any muscular response or guarding that one would otherwise expect to be present. The omentum, often referred to as the 'abdominal policeman', may be prevented by the enlarged uterus from moving to the site of inflammation, thus leading to unusual clinical picture. It is important to bear in mind the changing position of intra-abdominal organs at different gestational ages. For example, the appendix is located at the McBurney point in nonpregnant women and in early pregnancy. In the second trimester and thereafter, the appendix is progressively displaced upward and laterally, until it is closer to the gallbladder in late pregnancy.

During examination of the pregnant woman, the health of the fetus should also be assessed, which in early pregnancy means documentation of the presence or absence of fetal heart beat by Doppler or ultrasonography.

Pain from the uterus, cervix and adnexae are mediated through the tenth thoracic to first lumbar spinal nerves. The lower ileum, sigmoid colon and rectum share the same innervation and so differentiating between bowel and gynaecological pain is frequently problematic.

In addition, severe acute pain is often accompanied by nausea and vomiting, restlessness and sweating, owing to an autonomic reflex response to visceral ischaemia, inflammation or injury.

Clinical features

GENERAL EXAMINATION

A general survey can reveal important information such as anaemia (uterine or intra-abdominal haemorrhage), jaundice (pre-existing liver disease), cold and clammy limbs (hypotension, shock) or warm periphery (sepsis or pyrexia from any cause).

Tachycardia and hypotension is suggestive of haemorrhage, sepsis or torsion of adnexa. Pregnant women tend to be young and fit and can often maintain a normal blood pressure with increasing tachycardia until blood loss amounts to 30–35% of the total blood volume leading to decompensation and hypotension.

Fever and chill could be associated with intraperitoneal infection, torsion of the adnexa, cholecystitis, pyelonephritis and appendicitis.

GENITAL TRACT SIGNS AND SYMPTOMS

Vaginal bleeding is associated with complications of pregnancy, such as miscarriage and ectopic pregnancy. A foul-smelling discharge from the vagina can be caused by a septic miscarriage, ruptured membranes or genital tract infection. The cervical os may be open (inevitable, incomplete or septic miscarriage) or closed (missed or complete miscarriage) depending on the type of miscarriage.

In cases of septic miscarriage, there is usually a history of recent instrumentation of the uterus or attempts to induce miscarriage. Associated adnexal tenderness might represent pelvic inflammation.

PERITONEAL SIGNS

Abdominal rigidity and guarding, rebound tenderness, absence of bowel movement or expulsion of flatus, distended tympanitic percussion note and tenderness suggest peritonitis and may be present in case of bowel obstruction, inflammation or perforation. The patient tends to keep as still as possible to avoid pain on moving or coughing. These symptoms may also be a feature of intrabdominal bleed or infection due to ruptured ectopic gestation or septic abortion complicated by uterine perforation.

In addition, cervical excitation may accompany pelvic inflammation or infection associated with ruptured or twisted ovarian cyst and appendicitis. Rovsing's sign is classically described to be associated with appendicitis but this sign is usually absent in second half of pregnancy. This sign is positive when pressure on the left iliac fossa causes pain on the right.

OTHER GASTROINTESTINAL FEATURES

Diarrhoea, mucous discharge or bleeding from the rectum is often a manifestation of inflammatory bowel disease but can be present in pelvic abscess or haematoma from any cause. Irritation of the bowel by an infective, inflammatory agent or blood is thought to be the mechanism. Vomiting or nausea is common in acute pelvic pain but can often be dismissed as an early pregnancy symptom.

A rectal examination must be performed if any disease of the bowel is suspected.

RENAL TRACT SIGNS AND SYMPTOMS

Suprapubic discomfort, dysuria, frequency, urgency and haematuria are symptoms strongly suggestive of urinary tract infection. Restlessness may be a sign of urinary retention which is sometimes associated with a retroverted uterus, although this is uncommon in early pregnancy. Loin pain often radiating to the groin is a feature of renal or ureteric stone.

Investigations

Some commonly used laboratory tests have altered reference ranges in pregnancy. It is advisable to check with your individual laboratory about the normal ranges of test results applicable to gravid women. These changes can make the initial evaluation process somewhat difficult. For example, an inflammatory process such as appendicitis would be expected to produce an elevated white cell count, but pregnancy alone can produce white blood cell counts in the high normal range in the second and third trimesters and higher still in early labour.

Imaging in pelvic pain in pregnancy

ULTRASOUND

There are plenty of published reports which support the safety of ultrasound in pregnancy. Ultrasound is probably the most frequently used imaging modality for evaluating the abdomen and pelvis of a pregnant woman. Ultrasound is very useful in the diagnosis of following disorders:

- ectopic pregnancy
- miscarriage
- ovarian cyst haemorrhage
- ovarian cyst torsion
- fibroids
- cholecystitis
- appendicitis
- renal pathology.

It is also used with graded compression as a diagnostic aid in appendicitis.

The use of ultrasonography is essential for fetal evaluation. It helps to establish gestational age and fetal viability, to exclude congenital anomalies and to assess amniotic fluid volume and fetal wellbeing.

RADIOLOGY

Ionising radiation in the evaluation of pregnant women is often a source of anxiety for the practicing clinician but radiation exposure from a single diagnostic procedure does not result in harmful fetal effects. Table 7.1 shows the amount of radiation exposure to the fetus with some of the common radiological investigations.

Table 7.1 Radiation exposure of fetus – exposure depends on the number of films (from *Obstetrics and Gynecology Journal* 104 (3), ACOG Committee Opinion No. 299, Guidelines for Diagnostic Imaging During Pregnancy, 647–651, 2004. Reprinted with permission from Lippincott Williams & Wilkins)[1]

Procedure	Fetal exposure (1 rad = 0.01 Gy)
Chest radiographs (2 views)	0.02-0.07 mrad
Abdominal film (single view)	100 mrad
Intravenous pyelography	≥ 1 rad
Hip film (single view)	200 mrad
Mammography	7–20 mrad
Barium enema or small bowel series	2–4 rad
CT scan head or chest	< 1 rad
CT scan abdomen and lumbar spine	3.5 rad
CT pelvimetry	250 mrad

CT = computed tomography

During pregnancy, only medically indicated diagnostic radiograph procedures should be performed, but other imaging procedures not associated with ionising radiation should be considered instead of radiographs, when possible. If multiple diagnostic procedures are needed, it is reassuring to bear in mind that exposure to less than 0.05 Gy has not been associated with an increase in fetal anomalies or pregnancy loss. However, owing to the possible association of prenatal radiation exposure with childhood cancer, exposure to ionising radiation should be minimised when possible without compromising patient care.

MAGNETIC RESONANCE IMAGING

Magnetic resonance imaging (MRI) uses magnets rather than ionising radiation to alter the energy state of hydrogen protons. Although no adverse fetal effects have been documented, it is advisable that MRI should not be used in the first trimester. Not all MRI contrast agents are approved for use in pregnancy. Intravenous gadolinium crosses the placenta and the effects on the fetus are not understood. In some series, MRI was found to be useful in the diagnosis of acute appendicitis when ultrasonography was inconclusive.[2–5]

Management of abdominal and pelvic pain

The treatment of abdominopelvic pain depends on whether there is acute abdomen in pregnancy and on its specific cause. Emergency surgery for a pregnant woman should be performed for the same reasons as is applicable to the non-pregnant patient. If surgery is required but is considered elective, then it is prudent to wait until after the pregnancy is over. If surgery is required, an attempt should be made to postpone the procedure until the second trimester, if possible. The risk of preterm labour and delivery is lower in the second trimester compared with the third, and the risk of spontaneous loss and risks from medications such as anaesthetic agents are lower in the second trimester compared with the first.

GENERAL MANAGEMENT

Depending on the woman's condition the airway, breathing and circulation or ABC approach may be required for initial resuscitation together with assessment. Other measures may be required:

- Intravenous access is necessary if there has been a significant intravascular fluid loss secondary to haemorrhage, vomiting, pyrexia, bowel obstruction. At least two large-bore 16G cannulae should be sited.
- Intravenous fluids – infusion of crystalloids, colloids and blood should be considered to replace fluid depletion and blood lost due to any significant bleeding.
- Analgesia.
- Oxygen inhalation, where oxygen saturation is low or where the woman is dyspnoeic. If needed, a flow rate of 15 l/minute should be used.
- If there are features of sepsis, broad-spectrum antibiotics should be considered after samples for blood culture are taken.
- In a haemodynamically unstable patient, fluid intake and output should be monitored.
- Prophylactic low molecular weight heparin should be considered if a long period of restricted mobility is expected.

LAPAROSCOPY DURING PREGNANCY

In the past, laparoscopy during pregnancy was thought to be too risky to perform and most gynaecologists considered that it was contraindicated in pregnancy. However, following publication of multiple reports of successful use of diagnostic and therapeutic laparoscopy, this procedure has become increasingly popular in the treatment and evaluation of acute abdomen in pregnancy.[6–8] Although the safest entry technique for laparoscopy and optimal methods for maternal and fetal monitoring continue to be debated, it is accepted that laparoscopic surgery can be safely performed on pregnant women during any trimester, without any appreciable increased risk to the mother or fetus.[8–10] While the guidelines developed by the Society of American Gastrointestinal Endoscopic Surgeons suggest an open approach (Hasson technique) to entering the abdomen to avoid potential injury to the gravid uterus with the Veress needle or trocar, others have used a Veress needle to create pneumoperitoneum without any increase in maternal or fetal morbidity.[11,12] Carbon dioxide insufflation of 10–15 mmHg is considered safe. Owing to the carbon dioxide exchange in the peritoneal cavity and concerns over the effects of acidosis on the fetus, the use of capnography during laparoscopy in pregnant women is recommended.[11]

During laparoscopy, care must be taken to adjust the placement of the trocar based on uterine size, to minimise manipulation of uterus as much as possible and to keep surgical times as short as possible. Monitoring the fetal heart beat is useful but this is mostly impractical in the first trimester. The advantages of laparoscopy over laparotomy include shortened hospital stay, less need for analgesia, easier postoperative ambulation and earlier postoperative tolerance of oral intake.

Commonly encountered conditions causing abdomino-pelvic pain in early pregnancy

OVARIAN CYST ACCIDENTS

The reported incidence of ovarian cyst in pregnancy ranges from 1% to 25% and the routine use of ultrasound in pregnancy has significantly contributed to the high prevalence noted in recent literature.[13,14] Complications of ovarian cysts can be classified into three types: haemorrhage, rupture and torsion. All of these present with varying degrees of pain (Figure 7.1).

Table 7.2 shows clinical features associated with cyst accidents. These features are typical but not universal, as there is a wide variation in the clinical presentation of women with ovarian cyst accidents.

HAEMORRHAGE AND RUPTURE OF OVARIAN CYST

Haemorrhage into a corpus luteal cyst is probably the most common cause of unilateral pain in early pregnancy (Figures 7.2–4). The

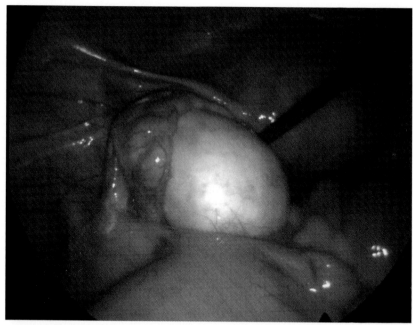

Figure 7.1 Dermoid cyst of left ovary in early pregnancy. This 6 x 6 x 5 cm cyst was impacted in the pouch of Douglas, causing pelvic pain; laparoscopic excision of cyst was performed

Table 7.2 Clinical features associated with cyst accidents (reprinted from *Best Practice and Research: Clinical Obstetrics and Gynaecology* 23 (4), Bottomley C and Bourne T, Diagnosing Miscarriage, 463–77, 2009, with permission from Elsevier)[4]

Feature	Haemorrhage/rupture	Torsion
Temperature	Normal or slightly raised	Raised in 10%, more likely if torsion occurred some hours previously
Pulse	Elevated	Significantly elevated
Blood pressure	Normal, unless massive haemorrhage into or from a cyst	Decreased if systemic disturbance from ischaemia and necrosis
Abdominal examination	Focalised or generalised tenderness	Generalised distension and peritonism
	Possible guarding or rebound tenderness	Possible loss of bowel sounds
Vaginal examination	Cervical excitation and adnexal tenderness	Cervical excitation and adnexal tenderness
	Possible cyst palpation	Possible adnexal mass palpable

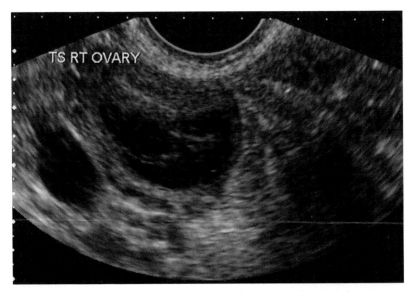

Figure 7.2 Transverse section of an ovary with haemorrhagic corpus luteum cyst; cross-section of right iliac vein is seen adjacent to the cyst

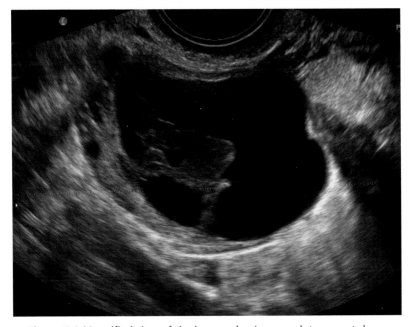

Figure 7.3 Magnified view of the haemorrhagic corpus luteum cyst shown in Figure 7.2 surrounded by normal ovarian tissue with follicles

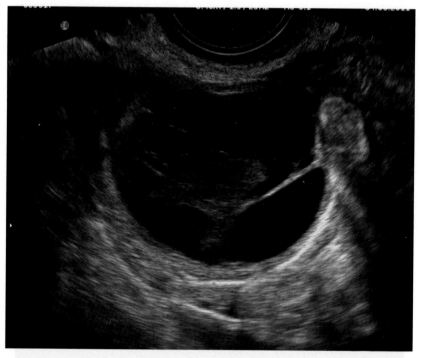

Figure 7.4 Magnified view of the haemorrhagic corpus luteum shown in Figure 7.2 demonstrating typical ultrasound scan features

mechanism of pain is thought to be stretching of the ovarian capsule. This condition should be managed conservatively unless clinical features necessitate surgical intervention.

Rupture of an ovarian cyst is rare but may occur spontaneously. Patients may give a history of mild trauma, such as caused by a fall, intercourse or vaginal examination. Commonly there is a recent history of chronic lower abdominal discomfort that has suddenly intensified. Where there is rupture of the cyst, blood in the pelvis can cause peritoneal irritation characterised by rebound and guarding and increased pain on movement. Significant blood loss will lead to hypovolaemic shock and in its early stages in healthy pregnant women the only manifestation may be tachycardia and postural hypotension.

The haemoglobin level may drop. In cases of cyst rupture, ultrasonography can help to detect the presence of fluid in the pouch of Douglas although a slight amount of fluid in the pelvis may be a physiological finding. Typical features of cyst haemorrhage are an ovarian cyst with mixed bizarre internal echoes reminiscent of a spider's web, suggestive of a blood clot. The clot may be seen to wobble like jelly on pressure from the vaginal probe.

Surgical treatment might become necessary and if so, the objective should be to conserve as much ovarian tissue as is safely possible. In the absence of malignancy, the prognosis is excellent.

TORSION OF THE ADNEXA

Adnexal torsion occurs when the ovary, often together with the adnexa or occasionally the fallopian tube on its own, twists or rotates partially or completely on its pedicle, resulting in venous obstruction in the initial stages and arterial obstruction later on. Adnexal torsion is unusual and occurs predominantly in teenagers and young women. Pregnancy predisposes to adnexal torsion with one in five such cases occurring during pregnancy.[15,16] The condition is associated with an ovarian mass in 50–60% of women and the mass is most often a dermoid cyst. Adnexal torsion occurs more frequently on the right side than on the left, by a ratio of three to two; this may be attributed to the physiologically longer ovarian ligament on the right side or to the presence of sigmoid colon on the left side limiting the space available for potential torsion.[17] Adnexal torsion occurs most frequently in the first trimester, occasionally in the second trimester and rarely in the third trimester.[16,18]

The woman may present with acute, severe colicky, unilateral lower abdominal and pelvic pain which usually arises from ischaemia and, often, necrosis of the ovary and adnexa. In addition systemic upset is common, such as anorexia, nausea and vomiting. A low-grade fever may be present. A tender adnexal mass may be palpable on bimanual pelvic examination.

The serum white cell count and C-reactive protein levels are often raised. Ultrasound scan features are of a unilateral enlarged oedematous ovary with peripheral follicles, with or without an ovarian cyst (Figure 7.5). Colour flow Doppler examination can detect absent ovarian blood flow in the central ovarian parenchyma.

Laparoscopy is helpful in confirming diagnosis as well as in surgical treatment. The aim should be to conserve as much ovarian tissue as possible. If the tissue is necrotic, removal is warranted and unilateral salpingo-oophorectomy is appropriate (Figure 7.6). If a partial torsion is confirmed, conservative management should be considered. If removal of the corpus luteum is necessary before 10 weeks of gestation, progesterone supplementation is necessary.

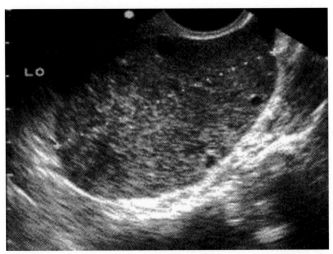

Figure 7.5 Transvaginal ultrasound scan showing an enlarged oedematous ovary with peripherally displaced follicles, suggestive of adnexal torsion (reprinted from *Best Practice and Research: Clinical Obstetrics and Gynaecology* 23 (5), Valentin L, Characterising actue gynaecological pathology with ultrasound, 577–593, 2009, with permission from Elsevier)

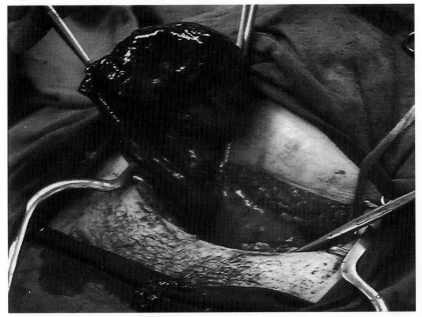

Figure 7.6 Torsion of the adnexa resulting in gangrenous right ovary and tube

UTERINE MYOMA

Red degeneration typically presents in the late first trimester and second trimester, which corresponds to the period of greatest fibroid growth. It occurs in 5–10% of pregnant women with myomas. Rapid growth of a fibroid results in decreased perfusion as growth outstrips its blood supply. This produces ischaemia and necrosis (degeneration). The classical features of fibroid degeneration are localised tenderness over the fibroid, nausea, vomiting, low-grade pyrexia and mild leucocytosis. Ultrasound findings describe necrotic fibroids as exhibiting mixed echogenicity with areas of echolucency in the central area of the fibroid.

Red degeneration is a self-limiting process and hence management involves rest, hydration and analgesia. Analgesia is provided by narcotic or anti-inflammatory agents. If indomethacin is used for pain relief its use is restricted to women at less than 32 weeks of gestation, because of its effects in causing oligohydramnios and partial constriction of the fetal ductus arteriosus. Prognosis is usually good.

URINARY TRACT INFECTION

Approximately 8% of women are diagnosed with urinary tract infection (UTI) in pregnancy.[19] There are three clinical manifestations of UTI in pregnancy:

- asymptomatic bacteriuria
- acute cystitis
- pyelonephritis.

Asymptomatic bacteriuria

Asymptomatic bacteriuria is significant bacteriuria without urinary symptoms. Treatment is important, as 30% of women will go on to develop acute cystitis.

Acute cystitis

Acute cystitis is characterised by dysuria, frequency, urgency, nocturia, haematuria, suprapubic discomfort with normal temperature and no systemic illness. A urine dipstick will show nitrites, leucocytes and blood. It is common to initiate empirical treatment and not wait for the results of urine culture and sensitivity. This will depend on local protocols and resistance in the local antenatal population. Treatment should be reviewed and changed if necessary once the results of culture and sensitivity are available. Treatment should be continued for at least 7–10 days. Follow-up is essential throughout the remainder of the pregnancy to ensure that it continues to be infection free.

Pyelonephritis

Pyelonephritis affects 2% of pregnant women. The early stages share the same clinical features as acute cystitis. In the later stages, systemic symptoms develop such as pyrexia, rigors, nausea, vomiting and renal angle pain. Serious sequel such as Gram-negative septicaemia and septic shock can occur. Investigations are outlined in Box 7.1 and include full blood count, CRP, renal function tests, blood cultures, urinalysis and urine culture and sensitivity. Treatment is usually as an inpatient with intravenous broad-spectrum antibiotics while waiting for the results of culture and sensitivities. It is important to evaluate response in 24–48 hours. Failure to improve may indicate a change of antibiotic or the presence of renal or ureteric calculi.

Further investigation of the renal tract with ultrasound may be necessary. Involvement of a urologist or renal physician should be considered and treatment usually includes analgesia, thromboprophylaxis and intravenous hydration if vomiting is a problem. Antibiotics should be given for at least 10–14 days. Urinary culture and sensitivity will need to be repeated throughout pregnancy to ensure absence of recurrence.

BOX 7.1 INVESTIGATIONS FOR PELVIC PAIN IN PREGNANCY AND ANY WOMAN IN THE REPRODUCTIVE AGE GROUP

- Urinary pregnancy test. Catheter specimen if the woman is unwell and unable to pass urine.
- Full blood count and depending on the clinical situation, urea and electrolytes, C-reactive protein, liver function tests, coagulation screen, group and save, blood culture.
- Urinalysis and urine culture and sensitivity if dipstick positive.
- Triple swabs.
- Arterial blood gases.
- Scan: transvaginal scan with or without transabdominal scan. Magnetic resonance imaging after first trimester.
- Laparoscopy may be the only way to diagnose or exclude pelvic pathology.

UROLITHIASIS

There may or may not be a previous history suggestive of urolithiasis. Pain is almost always the presenting symptom and this usually occurs in the flank. Dysuria, urgency, fever, nausea, vomiting and gross haematuria may be present. Costovertebral angle tenderness is a common feature.

Patients may have coexistent UTI. Microscopic haematuria is observed in 75% of cases. The absence of haematuria does not exclude a stone. Straining all urine samples is a simple and useful way to search for passage of stones with micturition. Ultrasound can reveal obstruction but physiological dilatation, usually of the right side in the second trimester, can produce false positive ultrasound images.

URINARY RETENTION

Urinary retention is commonly associated with impaction of a retroverted uterus in pregnancy. Predisposing factors include fibroids, uterine anomalies, adhesions and contracted pelvis. These can cause obstruction due to kinking of the urethrovesical junction or bilateral ureteric obstruction. Treatment is by catheterisation of the urethra until the uterus has enlarged and become an abdominal organ around 15 weeks of gestation.

APPENDICITIS

The incidence of appendicitis ranges from 1/1400 to 1/6000 deliveries. It is the most common non-obstetric cause of surgical emergency in pregnancy and seems to be more common in the second trimester.[20–24] Although the severity of appendicitis in pregnancy may be increased, the overall incidence is not affected by pregnancy. The incidence of perforation of appendix in pregnancy is 25%. If surgery for appendicitis is delayed to more than 24 hours the incidence of perforation increases to 66%.[25]

Pain is the most common presenting symptom and is located in the right lower quadrant in the first trimester. In the second trimester the appendix is located at the level of the umbilicus and the tenderness is located in the right periumbilical area or in the right upper quadrant. Nausea, vomiting and anorexia are other common features. Rebound tenderness and abdominal muscle rigidity is present in the majority of patients. Psoas irritation is observed less frequently during pregnancy compared with the nonpregnant state. Rectal tenderness is usually detectable in the first trimester. Fever and tachycardia are not sensitive signs.

The usefulness of white cell count in the investigation of appendicitis in pregnancy is limited. Severe disease can occur with a normal count. Polymorphonuclear leucocytes are often greater than 80% when appendicitis is present. In severe disease, an upright abdominal radiograph may show a right-sided mass or free air in the peritoneal cavity.

Most surgeons nowadays prefer appendicectomy by laparoscopic approach rather than through a laparotomy incision. Even if the appendix appears normal it should be removed because early disease may be present despite its grossly normal appearance and diagnostic confusion can be avoided in case of future recurrence of symptoms.

ACUTE CHOLECYSTITIS

Asymptomatic gall bladder disease is more common, occurring in 3-4% of pregnant women. The presenting symptom is usually right upper quadrant pain which may radiate to the back. Fever is unusual and vomiting is common. The right upper quadrant is tender to touch.

Gallstones are present in the vast majority of patients with acute cholecystitis. Leucocyte count and serum alkaline phosphatase are normally elevated. Aspartate transferase and alanine transferase may help to distinguish cholecystitis from hepatitis. Serum amylase levels might be elevated but a markedly elevated level is suggestive of pancreatitis.

Initial management is usually conservative in nature and usually includes intravenous fluid, analgesia and broad-spectrum antibiotics if symptoms persist and become systemic. It is important to bear in mind that analgesia with morphine may produce spasm of the sphincter of Oddi.

If conservative treatment does not produce symptom relief then surgery is indicated. Some surgeons favour early surgical intervention while others prefer to defer surgery to the postpartum period. There is evidence that laparoscopic cholecystectomy is safe in pregnancy. Laparoscopy can be safely performed in any trimester of pregnancy. A comparative study of conservative and surgical management of cholecystitis revealed the incidence of preterm delivery (3.5% and 6.0% respectively) and fetal mortality (2.2% and 1.2%). Fetal mortality in gallstone pancreatitis was 8.0% in a conservatively treated group of patients and 2.6% in a surgically treated group, suggesting that early surgical management is preferable.[26]

Following diagnosis of symptomatic cholelithiasis, the recurrence rate was 92% in the first trimester, 64% in the second trimester and 44% in the third trimester. Compared with patients who undergo cholecystectomy, patients in whom surgery is delayed experience increased hospitalisation, spontaneous miscarriage, preterm labour and preterm delivery. Fetal loss rates of 10–60% have been reported with gallstone pancreatitis.[11]

PANCREATITIS

Incidence of pancreatitis ranges from 1/1289 to 1/3333 deliveries. It is uncertain whether pregnancy predisposes to pancreatitis. Severe acute pancreatitis usually occurs in the third trimester of pregnancy and can result in significant maternal and fetal morbidity and mortality.[27] Cholelithiasis, alcohol use, hyperlipidemia, hyperparathyroidism, abdominal trauma and viral infection are risk factors for the development of pancreatitis. Of these risk factors, cholelithiasis is the most common in pregnant women with pancreatitis and is found in 90% of pregnancy-associated pancreatitis.[28–33]

Pregnant women present with similar clinical features as the nonpregnant patient. Abdominal pain, located in the epigastrium, is the most common symptom and onset is usually sudden. It is usually accompanied with nausea, vomiting and occasional low-grade fever. Jaundice may be seen. Epigastric tenderness is the most constant physical finding.

Serum amylase testing is most useful for diagnosis. During normal pregnancy, amylase levels may be slightly elevated but such elevation should be viewed with caution because they can occur with other disease entities such as intestinal perforation, infarction and intestinal obstruction. Other laboratory findings may include hyperglycaemia, hyperbilirubinaemia, hypocalcaemia, haemoconcentration and electrolyte imbalance. Sonography of the liver, gallbladder and pancreas may be helpful in confirming diagnosis.

Management of pancreatitis is usually conservative, including intravenous rehydration, correction of electrolyte, calcium and glucose imbalances. In the acute stage it is best to withhold oral feed and consider nasogastric suction. If gall bladder disease is causative, surgery can be performed when the patient's condition stabilises.

Acute symptoms last for approximately 1 week. The risk of perinatal mortality increases with the severity of the disease.

OVARIAN HYPERSTIMULATION SYNDROME

OHSS is an uncommon but potentially life-threatening complication of ovarian stimulation by ovulation induction agents. The majority of cases of severe OHSS are seen following in vitro fertilisation (IVF) treatment but the syndrome can occur after any form of supra-physiological ovarian stimulation, including clomifene and gonadotrophins. An accurate estimate of incidence of OHSS is difficult because of the variety of classification schemes used. About 33% of IVF cycles have been reported to be associated with mild forms of OHSS.[34] The severity of OHSS can worsen over time and even initially mild presentations should be kept under review. The incidence of OHSS is increased in young women, those with polycystic ovaries and in cycles where conception occurs, particularly multiple pregnancies.

Diagnosis of OHSS is usually straightforward given a history of ovarian stimulation, either by gonadotrophins or anti-estrogens, followed by typical symptoms of abdominal pain and distension, nausea and vomiting. Nevertheless, alternative diagnoses should always be considered as mentioned above.

OHSS is characterised by an increase in vascular permeability leading to a fluid shift from the intravascular to the extravascular space. This produces a reduction in circulating volume, depletion of albumin and electrolytes and third space accumulation of fluid manifest by ascites and, rarely, hydrothorax. This condition can be complicated by thromboembolism, renal failure, ovarian torsion, intra-abdominal bleeding, respiratory problems and acute respiratory distress syndrome, and hepatic dysfunction.

In addition to a full blood count, serum urea and electrolytes, liver function tests and clotting studies, pelvic ultrasound, chest X-ray, electrocardiogram and echocardiogram may become necessary.

The management of established OHSS should take place under the supervision of a specialist in reproductive medicine who is familiar with such disorders. There should be a low threshold for admission to hospital for adequate monitoring and treatment. Treatment includes correction of hypovolaemia with added potassium if necessary, prophylactic heparin, drainage of third space accumulation, if needed, and close monitoring of 'at risk' patients. Surgical intervention should be avoided. Pain relief is best provided with paracetamol or opiates. Nonsteroidal anti-inflammatory drugs are not recommended. Antiemetic drugs used should be those appropriate for the possibility of early pregnancy, such as prochlorperazine, metoclopramide and cyclizine.

Conclusion

Abdominal and pelvic pain in early pregnancy is common and diagnosis is often made difficult because many symptoms such as nausea, vomiting and pain are common in pregnancy. For any such case, the possibility of miscarriage and ectopic gestation should be considered at presentation. The decision for surgical intervention in early pregnancy should use the same criteria as for the non-pregnant woman, to reduce the risk of complications for the woman and fetus. Laparoscopy can be used safely in early pregnancy with consequent reduced recovery time.

Key points

- Women complaining of abdominal pain in early pregnancy as a result of non-obstetric causes are likely to present to early pregnancy assessment units.
- A multidisciplinary team approach must be considered in the management of these women because a wide range of differential diagnoses is possible.
- Emergency surgical intervention in a pregnant woman should be undertaken for the same indications as in a non-pregnant woman.
- Where indicated, laparoscopy can be safely undertaken in pregnancy by appropriately experienced personnel.

References

1. American College of Obstetricians and Gynecologists. *Guidelines for Diagnostic Imaging During Pregnancy*. ACOG Committee Opinion 158. Washington, DC: ACOG;1995.
2. Pedrosa I, Levine D, Eyvazzadeh AD, Siewert B, Ngo L, Rofsky NM. MR imaging evaluation of acute appendicitis in pregnancy. *Radiology* 2006;238:891–9.
3. Singh A, Danrad R, Hahn PF, Blake MA, Mueller PR, Novelline RA. MR imaging of the acute abdomen and pelvis: acute appendicitis and beyond. *Radiographics* 2007;27:1419–31.
4. Oto A, Ernst RD, Ghulmiyyah LM, Nishino TK, Hughes D, Chaljub G, et al. MR imaging in the triage of pregnant patients with acute abdominal and pelvic pain. *Abdom Imaging* 2009;34:243–50.
5. Singh AK, Desai H, Novelline RA. Emergency MRI of acute pelvic pain: MR protocol with no oral contrast. *Emerg Radiol* 2009;16:133–41.
6. Mazze RI, Kallen B. Reproductive outcome after anesthesia and operation during pregnancy: a registry study of 5405 cases. *Am J Obstet Gynecol* 1989;161:1178–85.
7. Gadacz TR, Talamini MA. Traditional versus laparoscopic cholecystectomy. *Am J Surg* 1991;161:336–8.
8. Rollins MD, Chan KJ, Price RR. Laparoscopy for appendicitis and cholelithiasis during pregnancy: a new standard of care. *Surg Endosc* 2004;18:237–41.
9. Affleck DG, Handrahan DL, Egger MJ, Proce RR. The laparoscopic management of appendicitis and cholelithiasis during pregnancy. *Am J Surg* 1999;178:523–9.
10. Sadot E, Telem DA, Arora M, Butala P, Nguyen SQ, Divino CM. Laparoscopy: a safe approach to appendicitis during pregnancy. *Surg Endosc* 2010;24:383–9.
11. Guidelines for laparoscopic surgery during pregnancy. Society of American Gastrointestinal Endoscopic Surgeons (SAGES). *Surg Endosc* 1998;12:189–90.
12. Lernaire BM, van Erp WF. Laparoscopic surgery during pregnancy. *Surg Endosc* 1997;11:15–8.
13. Booth RT. Ovarian tumors in pregnancy. *Obstet Gynecol* 1963;21:189.
14. Yazbek J, Salim R, Woelfer B, Aslam N, Lee CT, Jurkovic D. The value of ultrasound visualization of the ovaries durng the routine 11–14 weeks nuchal translucency scan. *Eur J Obstet Gynecol Reprod Biol* 2007;132:154–8.

15. Origoni M, Cavoretto P, Conti E, Ferrari A. Isolated tubal torsion in pregnancy. *Eur J Obstet Gynecol Reprod Biol* 2009;146:116–20.
16. Hibbard LT. Adnexal torsion. *Am J Obstet Gynecol* 1985;152:456–61.
17. Peña JE, Ufberg D, Cooney N, Denis AL. Usefulness of Doppler sonography in the diagnosis of ovarian torsion. *Fertil Steril* 2000;73:1047–50.
18. Huchon C, Fauconnier A. Adnexal torsion: a literature review. *Eur J Obstet Gynecol Reprod Biol* 2010;150:8–12.
19. McCormick T, Ashe RG, Kearney PM. Review: Urinary tract infection in pregnancy. *The Obstetrician and Gynaecologist* 2008;10:156–162.
20. Gomez A, Wood M. Acute appendicitis during pregnancy. *Am J Surg* 1979;137:180–3.
21. Horowitz MD, Gomez GA, Santiesteban R, Burkett G. Acute appendicitis during pregnancy. Diagnosis and management. *Arch Surg* 1985;120:1362–7.
22. Sivanesaratnam V. The acute abdomen and the obstetrician. *Baillieres Best Pract Res Clin Obstet Gynaecol* 2000;14(1):89–102.
23. Ankouz A, Ousadden A, Majdoub KI, Chouaib A, Maazaz K, Taleb KA. Simultaneous acute appendicitis and ectopic pregnancy. *J Emerg Trauma Shock* Jan 2009;2:46–7.
24. Hazebroek EJ, Boonstra O, van der Harst E. Concurrent tubal ectopic pregnancy and acute appendicitis. *J Minim Invasive Gynecol* 2008;15:97–8.
25. Jackson H, Granger S, Price R, Rollins M, Earle D, Richardson W. Diagnosis and laparoscopic treatment of surgical diseases during pregnancy: an evidence-based review. *Surg Endosc* 2008;22:1917–27.
26. Date RS, Kaushal M, Ramesh A. A review of the management of gallstone disease and its complications in pregnancy. *Am J Surg* 2008;196:599–608.
27. Sun L, Li W, Geng Y, Shen B, Li J. Acute pancreatitis in pregnancy. *Acta Obstet Gynecol Scand* 2011;90:671–6.
28. Wilkinson EJ. Acute pancreatitis in pregnancy: a review of 98 cases and a report of 8 new cases. *Obstet Gynecol Surv* 1973;28:281–303.
29. Ramin KD, Ramin SM, Richey SD, Cunningham FG. Acute pancreatitis in pregnancy. *Am J Obstet Gynecol* 1995;173:187–91.
30. DeVore GR. Acute abdominal pain in the pregnant patient due to pancreatitis, acute appendicitis, cholecystitis, or peptic ulcer disease. *Clin Perinatol* 1980;7:349–69.
31. Block P, Kelly TR. Management of gallstone pancreatitis during pregnancy and the postpartum period. *Surg Gynecol Obstet* 1989;168:426–8.
32. Kaiser R, Berk JE, Fridhandler L. Serum amylase changes during pregnancy. *Am J Obstet Gynecol* 1975;122:283–6.
33. McKay AJ, O'Neill J, Imrie CW. Pancreatitis, pregnancy and gallstones. *Br J Obstet Gynaecol* 1980;87:47–50.
34. Delvigne A, Rozenberg S. Epidemiology and prevention of ovarian hyperstimulation syndrome (OHSS): a review. *Hum Reprod Update* 2002;8:559–77.

8 Prescribing issues

Pregnancy, especially early pregnancy, is one of the most challenging situations in which clinicians prescribe medication. Fear of potential harm to the unborn is widespread among women as well as prescribers, leading to reluctance in both prescribing and compliance. However, it is vital to put the perceived teratogenic risks of medications into perspective with the risks of an untreated medical condition endangering maternal and fetal condition.

Approximately 2% of all pregnancies in the UK are associated with congenital anomalies and, while only a small minority of these are associated with administration of medicines in and around pregnancy, these, being potentially avoidable, constitute a crucial group. Almost 50% of all pregnant women are prescribed some form of medication other than a vitamin or nutrient supplement during pregnancy.[1]

The effect of a drug on pregnancy depends on various factors including the drug itself, the dose used, the time of exposure to the drug and presence of pre-existing maternal risk factors. Exposure to a toxin during the pre-embryonic phase (up to 17 days post-conception) when the cells are rapidly multiplying either results in a miscarriage owing to death of the embryo or survival of a fetus without any harmful consequences: the 'all or nothing' effect.[2] Exposure to a drug during the embryonic phase from 18 days to 8 weeks post-conception can result in permanent organ damage (teratogenicity) and this effect may be dose-dependent. Beyond 8 weeks, if the fetus is exposed to drugs, it is unlikely to result in significant organ damage, although certain subtle changes in the growing organs such as the brain, kidneys or gut, may go undetected until late in life. As the gestational age of exposure to a drug is the single most important determinant of the teratogenic potential, it becomes crucial to determine the correct gestational age of the fetus to be able to counsel about the potential risks involved (Figure 8.1).

Knowledge of basic embryology, as well as the physiological changes encountered in pregnancy, is vital to aid appropriate counselling. Pregnancy affects the pharmacokinetics of the drugs by altering the drug absorption, distribution, metabolism or excretion. All these

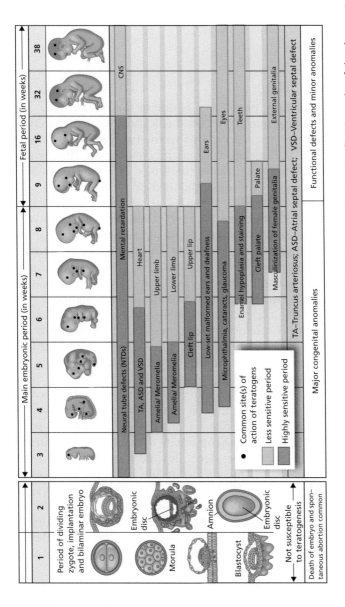

Figure 8.1 Schematic illustration of critical periods in human prenatal development. During the first 2 weeks of development, the embryo is usually not susceptible to teratogens; a teratogen either damages all or most of the cells, resulting in death of the embryo, or damages only a few cells, allowing the conceptus to recover and the embryo to develop without birth defects. Mauve denotes highly sensitive periods when major defects may be produced; green indicates stages that are less sensitive to teratogens when minor defects may be produced. (Reprinted from *The Developing Human: Clinically Oriented Embryology*, 8th ed. Moore KL and Persaud TVN, p. 182. Copyright Elsevier 2007)

changes may necessitate alteration of drug dosages in pregnancy.

Drug absorption may be affected by symptoms of nausea and vomiting in pregnancy, reduced gastric acid secretion and reduced gastrointestinal motility. Occasionally, compliance to a prescribed medication can be improved by simple measures like changing the time of the day when the drug is taken as, for some pregnant women, morning sickness may be a contributing factor for noncompliance.

Drug distribution in the body is altered owing to the increase in total body water and altered albumin concentrations. The metabolism of drugs may be affected by the circulating sex hormones in the pregnant state and may increase in the renal blood flow in pregnancy, resulting in altered plasma concentrations of drugs excreted in the urine.

Self-medication

Many women self-medicate with over-the-counter preparations and herbal remedies during pregnancy and consider these as safer. Women should be made aware of the fact that these preparations may be harmful for their pregnancy. Mild analgesics top the list of unprescribed medication taken and, while paracetamol is considered safe in pregnancy, the consumption of nonsteroidal anti-inflammatories such as ibuprofen can interfere with fetal renal function and may even precipitate premature closure of the ductus arteriosus.[3] Vitamin A in high doses is a known teratogen.

Prepregnancy counselling

Since most women attend for booking visit around 8–10 weeks of gestation, the majority of the vital organogenesis will have already occurred. Hence, it is ideal for women to have preconception counselling about the potential benefits versus risks of medication, including raising awareness of the reduction in the risk of developing neural tube defects by taking high-dose folic acid (5 mg) for at least 6 weeks prior to conception and continuing until the 12th week of gestation. Clinical condition permitting, non-essential drugs should be discontinued and appropriate medication with least teratogenic potential should be selected for treatment.

SAFETY OF DRUGS

Drugs with a good safety record in pregnancy include:

- analgesics such as paracetamol and opiates
- antacids
- antibiotics: penicillins, cephalosporins, clindamycin, erythromycin, nitrofurantoin (avoid near term)
- antihistamines
- corticosteroids
- laxatives
- insulin, thyroxine
- anti-hypertensives
- oral contraceptives (if used inadvertently in early pregnancy)
- antiviral medications: oral oseltamivir (Tamiflu®; Roche, Basel, Switzerland) or inhaled zanamivir (Relenza®; GlaxoSmithKline, Research Triangle Park, NC, USA).

Drugs potentially harmful in humans include:

- anti-epileptics: the most common congenital malformations associated with the intake of anti-epileptics, especially first-generation drugs such as phenytoin and phenobarbitone, are neural tube defects (spina bifida and hydrocephalus), cardiac and skeletal malformations and cleft lip and palate. Second-generation drugs such as sodium valproate and carbamazepine have also been associated with neural tube defects, with a quoted risk of about 2% for spina bifida with valproate and 1% with carbamazepine.[2] 'Fetal anticonvulsant syndrome', characterised by mid-facial abnormalities such as wide-spaced eyes, depressed nasal bridge, low-set ears and hypoplasia of distal digits has been associated with use of anti-epileptic drugs. The risk of malformations is high with polytherapy but there is not enough evidence to suggest that any particular combination is better than others. Based on data from the UK Registry, no major malformations were detected among 118 women exposed to a combination of carbamazepine and lamotrigine, while a combination of valproate and carbamazepine had a major malformation rate of 10% and combination of valproate with lamotrigine had a malformation rate of 9–12%.[2] Lamotrigine, although increasingly used for monotherapy, has been found to have a major malformation rate of 2.9% in the UK Registry, with a clear dose–response effect similar to valproate exposure.[2] Information on newer anti-epileptics such as levetiracetam is

limited but at high doses it is known to be associated with skeletal abnormalities and growth restriction in the fetus
- cytotoxic drugs
- lithium
- vitamin A
- warfarin
- danazol
- ACE-inhibitors.

In cases where drugs are thought to be associated with the congenital anomalies, a detailed ultrasound scan should be offered to check normality of the fetus (Table 8.1). The mother must be informed beforehand of the limitations of scanning and that functional abnormalities such as mental restriction are not detectable on ultrasound scan.

In the UK, a doctor is immune from civil liability for the adverse effects on the fetus of a drug appropriately prescribed in pregnancy if it is in line with established medical practice (Congenital Disabilities [Civil Liability] Act 1976). In situations where the clinician is

Table 8.1 Medications associated with specific congenital abnormalities (adapted from Rubin and Ramsay, *Prescribing in Pregnancy*, 4th ed., John Wiley & Sons)[2]

Fetal effect	Medication
Central nervous system, neural tube defects (spina bifida, anencephaly, encephalocele)	Sodium valproate, hydantoin, rifampicin
Structural defects	Retinoids, warfarin, carbamazepine, valproate
Cardiac	Lithium, thalidomide, retinoids, paroxetine, valproate
Renal (oliguria, renal failure)	NSAIDs, COX-2 inhibitors
Gastrointestinal tract (necrotising enterocolitis, gastroschisis)	Augmentin, NSAIDs, cannabis, recreational drugs
Facial (cleft lip and palate)	Rifampicin, retinoids, steroids, valproate benzodiazepines
Abnormal facial features	Alcohol
Skeletal	Thalidomide, cocaine, tetracyclines
Growth restriction	Beta blockers, alcohol, valproate, amphetamines
Placental abruption	Aspirin, warfarin, crack cocaine

confronted with having to offer advice to women who have inadvertently taken drugs for minor illnesses in pregnancy, it is best to base the advice on current information resources (Box 8.1).

Immunisations in pregnancy

Immunisation is only advisable in pregnancy if there is a clear indication and the benefits of immunisation clearly outweigh the risks. Generally speaking, live vaccines, such as BCG (Bacillus Calmette-Guérin), measles, mumps and rubella, yellow fever and oral polio preparations, should be avoided in pregnancy.

Pregnant women have been identified as a high-risk group for H1N1 viral influenza infection (swine flu). In view of the serious morbidity and mortality caused by swine flu in 2009, the Department of Health in UK modified its advice on seasonal flu vaccination in 2010/11 and now recommends all pregnant women be vaccinated with the trivalent seasonal influenza vaccine (which contains the influenza A/H1N1/ 2009-swine flu vaccine).[4] It is deemed safe to give seasonal influenza vaccine at any stage of pregnancy. Vaccination of pregnant women has been shown to be protective to the infant for the first 4–6 months of life through transfer of maternal antibodies.

Key points

- Check the pregnancy status in all women of childbearing age before prescribing.
- Drugs should be prescribed only when necessary. Where possible, non-drug measures should be tried first; for example, changes in diet for constipation.
- Counsel appropriately and, if feasible, before conception.
- The risks of not taking the drug on both maternal and fetal wellbeing must be balanced against the potential risks of the medication, if any.
- Use the lowest effective dose of the most suitable drug for the shortest possible duration.
- Choose a drug with the best safety record wherever possible.
- The majority of congenital anomalies are unrelated to drug use in pregnancy.
- Refer to appropriate sources for additional information.

References

1. Andrade SE, Gurwitz JH, Davis RL, Chan KA, Finkelstein JA, Fortman K, et al. Prescription drug use in pregnancy. *Am J Obstet Gynecol* 2004;191:398–407.
2. Rubin P, Ramsay M. *Prescribing in Pregnancy*. 4th ed. Oxford: Blackwell Publishing; 2008.
3. Welsh Medicines Resource Centre Prescribing in pregnancy. *WeMeReC Bulletin* 2000;7(3)1–5.
4. CMACE Emergent Theme Briefing 2 Maternal Mortality due to A/H1N1 2009 Influenza Virus, December 2010.

9   Ultrasound and screening

The main intentions of introducing the early pregnancy scan were to confirm viability of the gestation and to measure the fetal crown–rump length (CRL). However, in recent years, improvement in the resolution of ultrasound machines has made it possible to describe the normal anatomy of the fetus and to diagnose or suspect the presence of a wide range of fetal defects in the first trimester of pregnancy. Transvaginal ultrasonography (TVS) is widely used to assess early pregnancy and is considered to be safe for the developing embryo.

Visible signs of pregnancy

Around the time of implantation, a thickened hyperechogenic homogenous endometrium is detectable and is usually referred to as the 'decidual reaction'. A corpus luteum is usually seen in one of the ovaries showing a cystic or echogenic (haemorrhagic) pattern with typical peripheral blood flow resembling a 'ring of fire' on colour Doppler examination. The first visible sign of a definite pregnancy on TVS has been seen from days 28–31 with the appearance of the gestation sac, which appears as an uniform round hypoechoeic structure with an echogenic rim, asymmetrically situated within the decidua near the uterine fundus.[1,2]

At about 35 days, the secondary yolk sac makes its appearance and has developed from a layer of extra-embryonic endoderm and a layer of extra-embryonic mesoderm outside it. It is a spherical hyperechoic ring eccentrically situated within the gestation sac. The yolk sac increases in size until it begins to regress at around 9 weeks of gestation and usually disappears by 12 weeks.

The yolk sac is always seen by the end of the 6th week. The earliest embryonic pole has been reported to be visualised from day 35 and appears as a small linear echogenic structure adjacent to the yolk sac (Figure 9.1).[3] This appearance of the yolk sac and embryonic pole has been likened to a 'signet ring'. Since the connecting stalk is short, the embryonic pole is found near the wall. A heart pulsation is usually seen as soon as an embryonic pole is visualised but a normal outcome

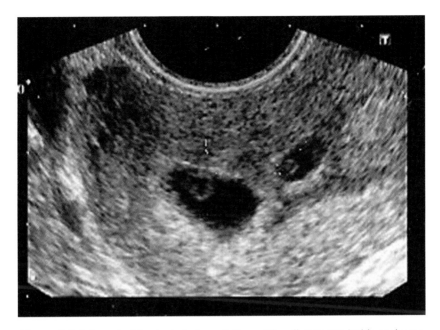

Figure 9.1 A 6-week dichorionic twin gestation with yolk sac seen inside each sac; a signet ring appearance is visible in the larger sac

should not be ruled out unless the embryo exceeds 6 mm in length. The embryo gradually becomes a 'kidney bean' shaped structure and is positioned further from the yolk sac, to which it is connected by the vitelline duct.

At the end of week 5, the heart rate is about 100 beats/minute and increases to 130 beats/minute by the end of 6th week. At 6 weeks, the amniotic cavity is seen surrounded by a thin membrane around the embryo.

At 7 weeks the hypoechogenic brain cavity can be identified. The cavity of diencephalon (future third ventricle) runs posteriorly. The heart can be recognised as a beating and bright structure below the embryonic head at 7 weeks. The umbilical cord is short and shows a large celomic cavity at its insertion where the primary intestinal loop can be identified. The first sign of herniation of the gut occurs during week 7 as a thickening of the cord and showing a slight echogenic area at the abdominal insertion. The amniotic cavity becomes visible at the beginning of week 7 and, over time, gradually expands as the fetus begins to produce urine, finally fusing with the chorionic membrane by the end of 12 weeks.

The CRL is 15–22 mm at 8 weeks. The cephalic and caudal ends can be distinguished by the visualisation of the diamond-shaped rhombencephalon (hind brain) at the cephalic end. The rhombencephalic cavity (future fourth ventricle) lies posteriorly and assumes a pyramidal shape. The mesencephalon lies at the top of the head. In some cases it is possible to recognise the fluid filled stomach as a small hypoechogenic area on the left side of the upper abdomen below the heart at the end of week eight.[4]

At 9 weeks, the fetus has a crown rump length of 23–31 mm. The bright choroid plexus of the lateral ventricles are regularly detectable at 9 weeks 4 days. The heart rate increases to a mean of 175 beats/minute.

From 8^{+3} weeks to 10^{+4} weeks of gestational age, all embryos have herniation of the midgut presenting as a large hyperechogenic mass. The stomach can be detected in 75% of the embryos before 10 weeks.

At 9 weeks (CRL 23–31 mm) it is possible to obtain recognisable image of the human body profile. The mouth and ventral body wall is well defined. The lateral ventricles and choroid plexus within are detectable at 9^{+4} weeks. The embryonic head is relatively large.

The embryonic phase is usually said to have ended at the end of 9 weeks. The fetal phase commences from 10 weeks when organogenesis is essentially complete and further development involves predominantly growth and organ maturation of the fetus until term.

During weeks 10 and 11 (CRL 32–54 mm) the fetal body elongates and the limbs, including the hands and feet, are recognisable. The fetal head is still relatively large with a prominent forehead and a flat occiput. The future skull can be distinguished, the ossification beginning at about 11 weeks with the occipital bone. At 10 weeks the moving heart valves and the interventricular septum can be identified. The heart rate slows down to 165 beats/minute at the end of week 11. The fetal midgut herniation retracts in to the abdominal cavity by the end of 12th week and the stomach bubble is visible in all fetuses by 11 weeks.

The dating scan

In the current practice of obstetrics, an accurate knowledge of the gestational age becomes necessary to plan interventions in pregnancy. Some examples are the appropriate timing of administration of antenatal steroids for fetal lung maturation, deciding whether tocolysis is necessary for threatened preterm labour and for satisfactory timing of elective induction of labour. The traditional method of relying on a woman's stated menstrual dates with supportive evidence from abdominal or vaginal examination, while reliable in most instances, may be inaccurate, especially when the date of the last menstrual period is uncertain or the menstrual cycle irregular. The estimated date of delivery (EDD) may be calculated by subtracting 3 months from the first day of the last menstrual period (LMP) and then adding one week and adjusting the year if necessary (Naegel's rule). However, even with apparently certain dates, menstrual age and ultrasound age of fetus were found to be discrepant in up to 45% of cases, probably owing to the variability in the length of the follicular phase of the cycle.[5]

Many studies have now shown that ultrasound-based estimation of EDD is a better predictor of spontaneous labour. Therefore, regardless of certainty and accuracy of date of LMP, a first-trimester scan should be used in all cases to date the pregnancy according to CRL. The LMP is useful only to guide the timing of the dating scan. This policy is supported by the National Institute for Health and Clinical Excellence (NICE), which recommends that all pregnant women be offered an ultrasound scan between 10 and 13 weeks of gestation to ensure consistency of gestational age assessments, improve the performance of mid-trimester serum screening for Down syndrome and reduce the need for induction of labour after 41 weeks. For women who present at or beyond 14 weeks of gestation, fetal head circumference or biparietal diameter is recommended for the estimation of gestational age, the former usually thought to be more accurate.

At 8 weeks of gestation the fetal head extends with lengthening and straightening of the torso, appearance of distinction between lower limbs and the 'rump' and hence the CRL can be measured which is around 18 mm at this stage. Towards the end of the first trimester, the CRL becomes technically more difficult to accurately measure because of movements, flexion and extension of the fetus. Ultrasound estimation of gestational age of fetus was first described by Robinson in 1973.[6] He used transabdominal scan between 6–14 weeks and showed that menstrual age could be predicted with 95% confidence intervals of around 4.7 days on a single measurement and 2.7 days if three independent measurements were taken of the same fetus. Many later studies using high resolution TVS have shown minimal variation in the findings of Robinson. For reasons mentioned above, the optimal time to date a pregnancy is said to be between 8 and 12 weeks. At this time the measurements are more accurate, consistently reproducible and prone to minimum variability as the growth of the fetus is greatest.[7]

Multiple gestation

Ultrasound plays an important role in the management of multiple pregnancies starting from the time of diagnosis and determination of chorionicity in early pregnancy up until the delivery of the second twin. Multiple pregnancy affects morbidity and mortality of both mother and fetus and therefore early diagnosis in the first trimester is important for planning of care and surveillance throughout pregnancy.

Ultrasound is not always accurate in determining zygosity but is very useful in determining placentation, which is more important in predicting the prognosis for twin pregnancy complications. Determination of placentation can be undertaken by characterisation of the dividing membrane, visualisation of placental mass and determination of fetal gender. A thin wispy membrane, which is often difficult to visualize, may be indicative of monochorionic placentation. A thicker, often layered membrane is more typical of dichorionic placentation. The measurement of membrane thickness is not as useful for determining chorionicity as the appearance of the membrane at its insertion onto the chorionic plate or fetal surface of the placenta. Where placental tissue appears to fill the triangular space between the membranes at the insertion into the placenta, called the lambda or 'twin peak' sign, then a fused dichorionic–diamniotic (DCDA) placentation is likely (Figure 9.2). Two separate and distinct placentae also indicate a DCDA twin gestation. Where the insertion of the dividing membrane into the chorionic plate of the placenta is like a 'T' junction then a monochorionic-diamniotic placentation is very likely. In multiple pregnancy, the dating scan also determines fetal number, amnionicity and chorionicity and is ideally performed in the first trimester when accuracy for chorionicity determination approaches 100%.[8]

Role of ultrasound in screening for aneuploidy

In the 1970s, only women aged 35 years and over or those with a previously affected pregnancy were offered the option of invasive prenatal diagnosis using amniocentesis or chorionic villus sampling (CVS). It is well known that the risk of trisomy 21 increases with maternal age. As a screening test, a fixed maternal age (for example, 35 years) has the advantage of being inexpensive and readily available but it has poor sensitivity and a low positive predictive value. Given that, in the UK, an increasing proportion of women conceive at a later stage of their reproductive life, the sensitivity of a 35-year maternal age cut-off has increased to 53% by the start of this millennium. This, however,

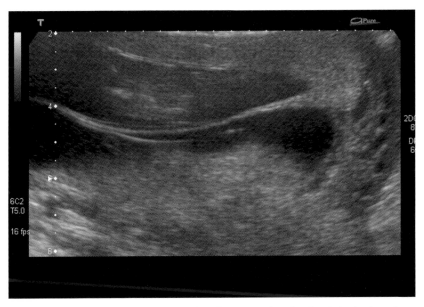

Figure 9.2 A dichorionic twin gestation demonstrating the 'lambda sign' on the right and a three-layer dividing membrane

is associated with a three-fold increase in the screen positive rate to 15%, which has significant implications in terms of pregnancy loss and financial cost.[9]

In subsequent years, various second-trimester screening tests became available, with the use of the biochemical markers alpha-fetoprotein (AFP), human chorionic gonadotrophin (hCG), unconjugated estriol and inhibin-A. The 'triple test' uses the first three markers and the 'quad test' uses all four. These screening tests are only available after 15 completed weeks of gestation, which means that prenatal diagnosis was only possible in the mid or late second trimester. Moreover, about 25% of Down syndrome cases are not detected with this screening approach and the false positive rate for these screening tests is approximately 5%.

In current day practice, owing to the need for earlier diagnosis, first-trimester screening methods have been implemented, using measurements of nuchal translucency (NT) alone and in combination with other sonographic and serum markers.

FETAL NUCHAL TRANSLUCENCY

Nuchal translucency is a normal finding and refers to the normal subcutaneous fluid-filled space between the back of the fetal neck and the overlying skin. This area can be sonographically measured accurately and reproducibly between 10 and 14 weeks of gestation (Figure 9.3). It is commonly believed that the larger the NT measurement, the greater its association with trisomy 21, other aneuploidies, major structural malformations and adverse pregnancy outcome. The aetiology of increased NT may be variable but the commonly held causes are fluid accumulation owing to fetal cardiovascular defects, abnormalities in extracellular matrix or abnormal or delayed development of the lymphatic system.

The optimal gestational age for measurement of fetal NT is 11^{+0} weeks to 13^{+6} weeks, which corresponds to a CRL of 45–84 mm. Accuracy of NT measurement is essential for an accurate estimation of risk. The risk calculation is performed on a computer database established by the Fetal Medicine Foundation, the software for which can be obtained following appropriate training and accreditation.

Prospective studies involving over 200 000 pregnancies, including 871 fetuses with trisomy 21, have demonstrated that increased NT can identify 77% of fetuses with trisomy 21 for a false positive rate of 4.2%.[9]

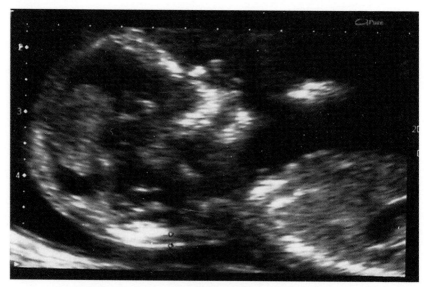

Figure 9.3 Fetal nasal bone; demonstrating calliper placement for measurement of nuchal translucency

FIRST-TRIMESTER COMBINED SCREENING TEST

In the presence of fetus with trisomy 21, maternal serum concentration of beta-hCG is increased and that of pregnancy-associated placental protein-A (PAPP-A) is decreased. In trisomies 18 and 13, maternal serum beta-hCG and PAPP-A are decreased. These fetoplacental biochemical markers have no significant association between fetal NT in either trisomy 21 or chromosomally normal pregnancies, so NT measurement and these serum markers can be combined to provide more effective screening than either method individually.

Many prospective screening studies have confirmed the feasibility and effectiveness of combining fetal NT and maternal serum free beta-hCG and PAPP-A in the detection of trisomy 21. One of these studies of 14 383 cases reported detection rates for fixed false positive rates of between 1% and 5% and false positive rates for fixed detection rates between 60% and 90% of screening for trisomy 21 by various different screening techniques. For a 5% false positive rate, the detection rate of trisomy 21 by the first-trimester combined test was 90%, which is superior to the 30% detection rate achieved by maternal age and 65% by second-trimester serum biochemistry.[9]

ABSENT NASAL BONE AND SCREENING FOR ANEUPLOIDY

Several studies have demonstrated a high association between absent nasal bone at gestational age of 11^{+0} to 13^{+6} weeks and trisomy 21, as well as other chromosomal abnormalities. In the combined data from these studies of a total of 15 822 fetuses, the fetal profile was successfully examined in 15 413 fetuses (97.4%). The nasal bone was absent in 176 of 12 652 (1.4%) chromosomally normal fetuses and in 274 of 397 (69%) fetuses with trisomy 21.[9] Similar to requirements of NT measurement, appropriate training and certification is necessary for ultrasound examination of fetal nasal bone.

In a case–control study of 100 trisomy 21 and 400 euploid singleton pregnancies, combining increased NT and absent nasal bone with maternal serum beta-hCG and PAPP-A at 11^{+0} to 13^{+6} weeks produced a detection rate of 97% for trisomy 21 for a false positive rate of 0.5%.[9]

Routine screening tests in early pregnancy

The following advice is based on guidance published by NICE.[10] For pregnant women who choose to have screening, the following tests need to be undertaken as appropriate:

- **blood tests** (ideally before 10 weeks): blood group, RhD status, screening for anaemia, haemoglobinopathies, hepatitis B virus, HIV, rubella susceptibility and syphilis
- **urine tests**: proteinuria and asymptomatic bacteriuria
- **ultrasound scan to determine gestational age**, using: (a) crown–rump measurement between 10^{+0} weeks and 13^{+6} weeks or (b) head circumference if crown–rump length is above 84 mm
- **Down syndrome screening**, using either: (a) combined test between 11^{+0} weeks and 13^{+6} weeks or (b) serum screening test, triple or quadruple, between 15^{+0} weeks and 20^{+0} weeks
- **ultrasound screening** for structural anomalies, normally between 18^{+0} weeks and 20^{+6} weeks.

ANAEMIA

In the UK, the normal range of haemoglobin in pregnant women up to 12 weeks should be at or above 11 g/dl and at 28–30 weeks of gestation, 10.5 g/dl. Haemoglobin levels outside the normal UK range for pregnancy should be investigated and iron supplementation considered if indicated. The cause of anaemia can be diverse; for example, iron deficiency, thalassaemia, sickle cell anaemia, and so the use of haemoglobin as the sole means of diagnosing anaemia is not a sensitive test, although this is often used as the first indicator in clinical practice. The impact of gestational age on the change in plasma volume must be considered while making a diagnosis of iron deficiency anaemia. Suspicion of iron deficiency anaemia should lead to serum ferritin estimation, which is the most sensitive single screening test to detect iron stores. Using a cut-off point of 30 micrograms/litre, a sensitivity of 90% has been reported.

BLOOD GROUP AND RED CELL ALLOANTIBODIES

All pregnant women, irrespective of their rhesus D status, should be offered screening for blood group and red cell alloantibodies. Women with clinically significant atypical red cell alloantibodies should be offered referral to a specialist for further investigation and advice on subsequent antenatal management. For women who are RhD-negative, consideration should be given to offering partner testing to determine whether the administration of anti-D prophylaxis is necessary.

HAEMOGLOBINOPATHIES

Preconception counselling and carrier testing about sickle cell anaemia and thalassaemia should be available to all women who are identified as being at higher risk of haemoglobinopathies, using the Family Origin Questionnaire from the NHS Antenatal and Newborn Screening Programme. The type of screening depends upon prevalence and can be carried out in either primary or secondary care. In high-prevalence areas, laboratory screening, preferably by high-performance liquid chromatography, should be offered to identify carriers of sickle cell disease and thalassaemia. If the woman is identified as a carrier of a clinically significant haemoglobinopathy, the father of the baby should be offered counselling and appropriate screening without delay.

SCREENING FOR INFECTION

Routine screening for asymptomatic bacteriuria by midstream urine culture early in pregnancy, identification of cases and their treatment reduces the risk of pyelonephritis.

Serological screening for hepatitis B should be offered to all pregnant women so that effective postnatal intervention can be offered to infected women to decrease the risk of mother to child transmission.

Detection and appropriate antenatal interventions for HIV infection in the mother can reduce mother to child transmission of HIV infection.

Identification of those pregnant women susceptible to rubella enables vaccination in the postnatal period for the protection of future pregnancies.

Screening for syphilis should be offered to all pregnant women at an early stage because treatment of syphilis is beneficial to the mother and baby.

Key points

- A high-resolution ultrasound scan in early pregnancy plays an essential role in planning management in later pregnancy.
- Screening for aneuploidy involves use of high-resolution ultrasound scanning in early pregnancy.
- Routine tests offered in early pregnancy help to exclude some common disorders.

References

1.   Warren WB, Timor-Tritsch I, Peisner DB, Raju S, Rosen MG. Dating the early pregnancy by sequential appearance of embryonic structures. *Am J Obstet Gynecol* 1989;161:747–53.
2.   Timor-Tritsch IE, Farine D, Rosen MC. A close look at early embryonic development with the high frequency transvaginal transducer. *Am J Obstet Gynecol* 1988;159:676–81.
3.   Britten S, Soenksen DM, Bustillo M, Coulam CB. Very early (24–56 days from last menstrual period) embryonic heart rate in normal pregnancies. *Hum Reprod* 1994;9:2424–6.
4.   Blaas Harm-Gerd, Eik-Nes S. Normal first trimester ultrasound findings. In: Nicolaides KH, Snijders RJM, Sebire N, editors. *The 11–14 Week Scan*. Diploma in Fetal Medicine Series. London: Informa Healthcare; 1999. p. 115–22.
5.   Gardosi J, Vanner T, Francis A. Gestational age and induction of labour for prolonged pregnancy. *Br J Obstet Gynaecol* 1997;104:792–7.
6.   Robinson H, Fleming JE. A critical evaluation of sonar crown–rump length measurements. *Br J Obstet Gynaecol* 1975;82:702–10.
7.   Nicholas M, Morgan E, Jensen JT. Comparing bimanual pelvic examination to ultrasound measurement for assessment of gestational age in the first trimester of pregnancy. *J Reprod Med* 2002:47:825–8.
8.   Carlin A, Neilson JP. Twin clinics: a model for antenatal care in multiple gestations. In: Kilby M, Baker P, Critchley H, Field D, editors. *Multiple Pregnancy*. London: RCOG Press; 2006. p. 121–38.
9.   Hyett J, Nicolaides K. First trimester ultrasound screening with nuchal translucency. In: Evans MI, Johnson MP, Yaron Y, Drugan A, editors. *Prenatal Diagnosis*. London: McGraw-Hill; 2006. p. 289–341.
10. National Institute for Health and Clinical Excellence. *Antenatal Care: Routine Care for the Healthy Pregnant Woman*. Clinical Guideline CG62. London: RCOG Press; 2008 [http://guidance.nice.org.uk/CG62/Guidance/pdf/English].

Further reading

Blackburn S. *Maternal, Fetal and Neonatal Physiology*. 3rd ed. London: Elsevier-Saunders; 2007.

Centre for Maternal and Child Enquiries. Saving Mothers' Lives: reviewing maternal deaths to make motherhood safer: 2006–08. The Eighth Report on Confidential Enquiries into Maternal Deaths in the United Kingdom. *BJOG* 2011;118 Suppl 1:1–203.

Edmonds DK, editor. *Dewhurst's Textbook of Obstetrics and Gynaecology*. 7th ed. Oxford: Wiley-Blackwell; 2007.

Farquharson RG, Stephenson MD, editors. *Early Pregnancy*. Cambridge: Cambridge University Press; 2010.

Heffner LJ, Schust DJ. *The Reproductive System at a Glance*. 3rd ed. Oxford: Wiley-Blackwell; 2010.

Luesley DM, Baker PN, editors. *Obstetrics and Gynaecology: An evidence-based text for the MRCOG*. 2nd ed. London: Hodder Arnold; 2010.

Rubin P, Ramsay M, editors. *Prescribing in Pregnancy*. 4th ed. Oxford: Wiley-Blackwell; 2007.

Schoenwolf GC, Bleyl SB, Brauer PR, Francis-West PH. *Larsen's Human Embryology*. 4th ed. Edinburgh: Churchill Livingstone; 2009.

Stables D, Rankin J. *Physiology in Childbearing*. 3rd ed. London: Bailliere Tindall Elsevier; 2010.

Index

Intrapartum Care for the MRCOG and Beyond (2nd edition)

This book provides a comprehensive overview of clinical intrapartum care. The emphasis is on a pragmatic approach which promotes the necessary vigilant care while also supporting the wishes of the woman who wants minimal interference. The content has been thoroughly updated to reflect current practice and developments in the field since the publication of the original edition.

This book is an invaluable aid, not only for candidates preparing for the Part 2 MRCOG examination, but also for those in clinical practice who want an update in the field, midwives and any health professional who comes into contact with mothers.

Contents: Improving intrapartum care; First stage of labour; Second stage of labour; Fetal surveillance in labour; Third stage of labour; Lower genital tract trauma; Induction of labour; Preterm labour and prelabour rupture of membranes; Assisted vaginal delivery; Shoulder dystocia; Breech vaginal delivery; Twin and triplet delivery; Caesarean section; Vaginal birth after caesarean section; Uterine rupture; Emergency obstetric hysterectomy; Cord prolapse; Antepartum haemorrhage; Postpartum haemorrhage; Acute uterine inversion; Amniotic fluid embolism; Disseminated intravascular coagulation; Acute tocolysis; Severe pre-eclampsia and eclampsia; Neonatal resuscitation; Perinatal loss.

ISBN: 9781906985400   295 pages   Published 2011

Fetal Medicine for the MRCOG and Beyond (2nd edition)

A solid understanding of fetal medicine is essential for the practice of obstetrics and gynaecology. This comprehensive book, which has been extensively updated to reflect current clinical practice and developments in the field since the original edition, is a vital source of information for both aspiring specialists and established practitioners.

This book will be of great assistance not only for candidates in their preparation for the MRCOG Part Two examination but also to anyone working in fetal medicine who wants to update their knowledge at any stage in their career. It will be an invaluable resource for any health professional who comes into contact with mothers and babies, including consultants, trainees and midwives.

Contents: Screening for chromosomal abnormalities; Prenatal diagnostic techniques; The routine anomaly scan; Fetal structural abnormalities; Fetal therapy; Prenatal diagnosis and management of non-immune hydrops fetalis; Termination of pregnancy for fetal abnormality; Fetal growth restriction; Twin pregnancy; Fetal infection.

ISBN: 9781906985363   214 pages   Published 2011

Gynaecological Oncology for the MRCOG and Beyond (2nd edition)

This book will be useful to those preparing for MRCOG Part 2, to those undertaking the ATSM in Gynaecological Oncology as well as proving a valuable resource for all those involved in the care of women with gynaecological cancer. It includes updated information on developments in care and presents the latest evidence on investigation, staging and management as well as new chapters focusing on the multidisciplinary approach.

Contents: Basic epidemiology; Basic pathology of gynaecological cancer; Preinvasive disease of the lower genital tract; Radiological assessment; Surgical principles; Role of laparoscopic surgery; Radiotherapy: principles and applications; Chemotherapy: principles and applications; Ovarian cancer standards of care; Endometrial cancer standards of care; Cervical cancer standards of care; Vulval cancer standards of care; Uncommon gynaecological cancers; Palliative care; Emergencies and treatment-related complications in gynaecological oncology.

ISBN: 9781906985219   261 pages   Published 2010

Gynaecological and Obstetric Pathology for the MRCOG and Beyond (2nd edition)

This book is an essential guide to practising gynaecologists dealing with the complexities of gynaecological and obstetric histopathology. It will also aid serious examination candidates by building a solid understanding of the subject where it relates to both gynaecology and obstetrics. It provides a newly revised, concise text and many helpful colour illustrations and is an excellent knowledge source and guide to revision, written by experts in the field.

Each subject area is conveniently organised around the relevant anatomical structures, with extensive and up-to-date coverage of both major and minor changes in gynaecological pathology since the publication of the first edition. No library should be without this concise, colourful text.

Contents: The vulva; The vagina; The cervix; The endometrium; The myometrium; The fallopian tube and broad ligament; The ovary; Abnormalities related to pregnancy; Cervical and gynaecological cytology.

ISBN: 9781904752769   238 pages   Published 2009

Paediatric and Adolescent Gynaecology for the MRCOG and Beyond (2nd edition)

Paediatric and adolescent gynaecology adds an interesting dimension to the spectrum of work for gynaecologists but can be intimidating. This concise book lays out the fundamentals of both investigation and management of the child, thereby enhancing confidence.

Updated by Professor Anne Garden, a recognised authority in the field, this edition includes an important chapter on child sexual abuse – a situation in which it is vital to do the right thing for the sake of the child.

The book is easy to read and makes a handy reference source for the MRCOG candidate. It is also likely to be kept close at hand to refresh the memory of the established practitioner intermittently encountering the younger patient.

Contents: Pubertal growth and development; Indeterminate genitalia; Gynaecological problems in childhood; Endocrine disorders; Child sexual abuse; Amenorrhoea; Menstrual problems in teenagers; Contraception; Female genital mutilation; Gynaecological tumours.

ISBN: 9781904752585   114 pages   Published 2008